THE
NEW WAY
TO EAT

Books by Linda Clark

Stay Young Longer
Get Well Naturally
Secrets of Health and Beauty
Help Yourself to Health
  (an ESP book)
Know Your Nutrition
Be Slim AND Healthy
Face Improvement
  Through Exercise and
  Nutrition
Are You Radioactive?
  How To Protect Yourself
The Best of Linda Clark
  An Anthology
The Linda Clark Cookbook

Rejuvenation
Color Therapy
Health, Youth and Beauty
  Through Color Breathing
  (with Yvonne Martine)
Beauty Questions and Answers
  (with Karen Kelly)
Handbook of Natural Remedies
  for Common Ailments
Health and Beauty for Your Pets
  Through Nutrition
How To Improve Your Health
  The Wholistic Approach to
  Health

NOTE: Due to an increasing number of letters and requests for information Linda Clark can no longer answer personal letters. She is not legally allowed to prescribe, recommend or advise on individual problems. She can, however, report on research which is available in her books, articles, scientific journals and elsewhere.

If you have further questions about information in connection with this book, please send them immediately to Good Health Keeping, P.O. Box 2614, La Mesa, California 92041. Questions of a general nature will be answered in a future publication.

THE
NEW WAY
TO EAT

Linda Clark

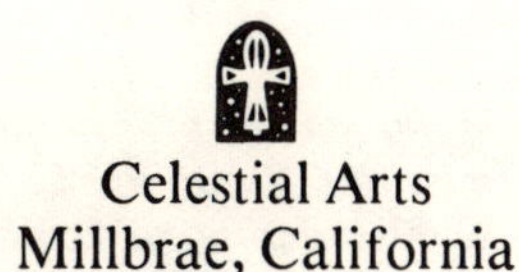

Celestial Arts
Millbrae, California

Parts of this book were derived from articles published in Let's LIVE Magazine.

Cover Design by Betsy Bruno

Celestial Arts
231 Adrian Road
Millbrae, California 94030

First Printing. March 1980
Made in the United States of America

Library of Congress Cataloging in Publication Data
Clark, Linda A.
      The new way to eat.

      Includes index.
      1. Nutrition.   2. Health.   I. Title.
QP141.C58   64.1   79-55271
ISBN 0-89087-263-5

1 2 3 4 5 6 7 — 86 85 84 83 82 81 80

The author wishes to gratefully acknowledge that a major portion of the information in this book is based on research presented by Weston A. Price, D.D.S. in his book, Nutrition and Physical Degeneration *with the permission of the publisher, Price-Pottenger Nutrition Foundation.*

Special thanks also goes to Pat Connolly, Curator of the PPNF for her patient and untiring dedication and for her permission to excerpt from her publication, A Guide to Living Foods *in which she shares her excellent recipes based on Dr. Price's research. (Also available at the address below.)*

Except for a few libraries and health stores, Dr. Price's book, Nutrition and Physical Degeneration, *is available only from the Price-Pottenger Nutrition Foundation, P.O. Box 2614, La Mesa, California, 92041. It is published only in hardcover, due in part to the importance of the clarity of the photographs (some of which have been reproduced here with permission). It contains 527 pages, 134 photographs and is available for $20.50 plus $2.00 shipping charge and sales tax for California residents.*

CONTENTS

CHAPTER ONE

Looking for Help

People are extremely confused these days about what to eat or what not to eat. The message about junk food has finally been accepted, but many people do not yet know what is and what is not a junk food.

To make matters worse, those who are just learning about nutrition are often being told by product commercials, "Take this vitamin, or this mineral and feel good!"

Unfortunately nutrition is not that simple. A single vitamin or mineral alone can't make you well, unless you are already well and are possibly deficient in that one element only. In nature, *all the nutrients occur together,* and if a person is deficient in one, he/she is usually deficient in many. So it is wiser, at least at first, to take the overall approach.

The late famed nutritionist, Dr. Royal Lee, stated, "Most people are willing to admit that the foundation of health is nutrition, and that most of our ill health of today is due to direct result of under-nutrition...

"The best chance we have of supplying our bodies with what they need is to eat the basic natural foods as originally intended . . .

"Will changing the diet actually restore health? Yes, it is possible, even probable. From the moment that your body begins receiving what nature intended it to have, restoration begins and age makes no difference. Many people who have been sickly and ailing at 60 years of age have, by changing their eating habits, produced a vital health picture at 80 . . ."[1]

If certain serious deficiencies have developed, taking vitamin/mineral supplements may be necessary either at first until a balance is restored or on a continuing basis, if the individual has a genetic assimilation problem for some nutrients.

This book is being written to help you choose the right things for *you* (we are all different, as our fingerprints, blood types, and so on, prove). Therefore you may need certain additional nutrients which your husband, wife, mother, father, sister or brother or child might not need at all.

A letter which came from a reader started the idea for this book on how to eat to help your health. The woman who wrote the letter was floundering, as you will see. She wrote:

Dear Linda Clark:

"I am at my wits end! For years I have had an external infection which will not clear up. I have gone from doctor to doctor and have swallowed pills and used creams until I have developed what I feel are additional skin problems directly related to the medicine I was using.

"I have also been to a dermatologist who prescribed cortisone cream for surface application, but this is apparently not the source of my problem (which seems to be more internally caused).

"As a result of conventional, orthodox treatment failing to cure the infection, and a subsequent skin rash plus dry, flaky skin on my scalp, I am desperate and frightened because as a result of my experiences I now have no confidence in the usual practitioner who uses drug therapy.

"I realize something is wrong and I have been trying nutrition on my own but can't seem to figure out by myself what vitamins/minerals to take. When I take the oily based vitamins (A, D and E) which I am sure I must need, I become violently nauseated.

"I have read your helpful book, *Know Your Nutrition,* which explains what each nutrient does, but I do not know *how much* to take.

"I have read about hypoglycemia and have all the symptoms.

"I smoke about two packages of cigarettes daily, drink one to two cups of coffee but am unable to tolerate the taste of tea.

"I am thirty-one years old, was one of fourteen children, all of whom were vitamin deficient as children. We all had the usual childhood diseases and even some adult diseases. My mother's side of the family has lived close to the one hundred mark; my father's side to approximately sixty. They had the usual adult ailments but for the most part seemed to recover.

"I have been medically tested, X rayed, probed and even hospitalized for a week for observation and the verdict has been that I am in relatively fine shape by medical standards. If so, why don't I feel better? I am so depressed and want desperately to get well. It is even affecting my psychological reactions, to the point that I dislike going out in public, though I am not housebound.

"I realize that not being a doctor, you cannot prescribe, but can you point the way towards a hopeful, helpful nutritional regime to help me improve my health and well-being?

"Please do help me in any way you can by showing me how to help myself. I don't want to be sick any more. Anything you suggest will be greatly appreciated."

C. W.
Illinois

I quote her with permission, though to protect her privacy, I have omitted her name. There was much more personal information in this letter, too long to reproduce here, but the message is clear: it is a cry for help which is the rule, not the exception, today. The symptoms may vary from person to person, but there is no doubt a common denominator underlying many different symptoms of various people. A doctor, after reading this letter might say, "Go to a psychiatrist!"

Unfortunately this has been tried many times before and though helpful in some cases, if there is a mental-emotional problem, couldn't it also be due to an out-of-tune body? We will discuss some new, exciting research in this area in Chapter Thirteen. The mind and emotions are all part of the same physical body, and in the opinions of nutritionists, experience has often shown that when the body chemistry is corrected, the mental-emotional symptoms are corrected too.

So perhaps this woman is right: the nutritional route may help her as it has helped so many others. It is at least worth a try. This woman, as her letter shows, is intelligent, thus wants some intelligent guidance in the nutritional field.

For this reason, I agreed to look for and provide some research which perhaps may help her problems, and hopefully, some problems of others as well, *if* the cause is due to nutritional deficiencies which is often the case.

In the pages which follow, you will *not* find the usual information which is repeated from book to book, article to article, which is the opinion of a single person. Instead there are some unique findings which have applied to the good health of many thousands that you may never have read before or maybe never thought of. If you wish to be healthier I believe the material is at least worth reading to learn how other people have bypassed the ailment route, though it may differ from that of the next person. (I hope you will find it as interesting as I did.) In addition, I hope you will learn something new and that you will be helped in some way. Perhaps completely, who knows? After all, health is probably your most priceless possession. Don't we all need to learn everything available to maintain it as well as how to prevent further illnesses?

This book should help!

NOTES

1. Royal Lee, D.D.S., "The Human Machine—Its Care and Repair," *Let's LIVE* Magazine 1968.

CHAPTER TWO

Can Food Really Affect Your Health?

It is true that you are, generally speaking, what you eat. Food is your body's fuel and the body machinery reflects, to a great extent, the kind of fuel you feed it. This applies to animals and plants as well. So health depends largely on what occurs in or is omitted from your diet. Many people insist it is your genes or your inheritance only which affects your health. You have heard the statement, "If you want to be healthy, pick a good set of parents." This may be true but it also follows that what your parents, or *their* parents, or the generations before them ate, affected them, which in turn has affected you. Your diet will also affect your own children. Genes are biological factors which can be influenced by nutrition, good or bad. So we come full circle.

Take birth defects as an example. For years the cause of birth defects was a mystery before it became clear that what the mother and father ate before conception and what the mother ate during pregnancy was a clue. If the diet was inadequate, the nutritional building blocks needed to make a whole and healthy baby were also inadequate. One well-known nutritionist, when asked why he wore glasses in spite of his super diet, explained that his vision problems could be traced to his mother's inadequate diet. Another example: babies, with alcohol on their breath, have been born of alcoholic mothers.

I have inherited problems in the same way. My mother was proud of her diet. And measured by money, it was probably considered above average. Yet she began to eat white bread which was stripped of wheat germ and vitamin E around the turn of the century and I paid the consequences with my own health by being born with a vitamin E deficiency.

At that time there was a fetish about food being "pure white" and sterile. The whole brown, natural flour was not only made white by stripping, but in some areas, (fortunately not in mine) bleach was added to make it still whiter. This bleach gave dogs convulsions and it took a long time for manufacturers to realize its danger for humans. However, they found that denuding the flour did help to make it last longer on the grocery shelf without spoilage, and thus saved money for millers and grocers. So commercial pressures made it fashionable to use white flour exclusively. My mother used to tell me proudly how her mother made her own "beautiful" white bread and rolls. By the time she learned of the value of nutritious whole grain flour and bread, it was too late for me. The vitamin E flour robbery had already occurred.

It was not until years later that the resulting damage for the majority was discovered. First, cattle, though appearing normal, began dropping dead of heart attacks. The cause was finally found to be the lack of wheat germ which contains vitamin E, now considered a heart-protective vitamin. This valuable substance had been omitted from grains as well as the cattle feed. When it was restored to cattle feed, the heart attacks and deaths in the animals ceased.[1]

But still more important, humans began following suit, although doctors did not recognize the cause then, nor do many of them realize it now. But Wilfrid E. Shute, M.D., the heart and vitamin E specialist, stated in connection with the vitamin E robbery at the turn of the century, "Prior to the removal of the wheat germ with its vitamin E from the flour, *there were no cases of coronary thrombosis. Now it is one of the nation's major killers.*[2] (Italics mine.) At the time of the vitamin E robbery, this was an exception, since it was the only vitamin known to be deliberately removed from our food. Today nutritional food robbery is no longer an exception, but the rule. Much of our food is taken apart and put back together again, either omitting or damaging fragile vitamins and minerals. Why? The food processors claim it is because the public wants it this way: that they (the public) want convenience foods like TV dinners; that they want food to taste and look more *natural.* So the manufacturers add artificial colors, which have been found to cause cancer, to brighten up the food; they add unsafe chemicals to enhance taste; and they claim they want to protect food against spoilage, which is accomplished by adding questionable preservatives. Food tampering is common.

An example is honey, which nutritionists believe should be eaten raw to provide all available nutrients, particularly those damaged by heat. But on the grocery shelves you will usually find a jar of honey marked "Super, Deluxe" which is heated, strained and so clear you can read the back of the label through it. It is also more expensive. Natural honey, with its important nutrients, should be unheated and slightly cloudy. So the public pays twice for these so-called refined foods: they pay the grocer, then on eventually acquiring nutritional deficiency ailments from overprocessed foods, they pay the doctor to try to patch them up again.

Unfortunately, doctors are not taught nutrition in medical schools, but mainly surgery and the use of drugs which usually have temporary effects, whereas nutrition helps to rebuild the body. Doctors usually tell their patients just to eat a good diet and they will get everything they need. *This is not true today!* It was true at one time however, and there are reports, complete with photographs, to prove that whole natural food could and did produce glowing health.

Although anthropologists have studied this subject of health versus diet for years, reports did not always reach the public, at least in an easily understood manner. So it was a relief to learn that one man has done an in-depth study which he presented in an easy-to-read book, complete with hundreds of photographs. This man, Dr. Weston A. Price, a dentist, set out on a world tour to visit at least fourteen primitive tribes, observe their teeth and health and examine their diet. He found and proved with pictures (which do not lie) that there was, indeed, a close connection between good teeth, good health and good food. The name of his book is *Nutrition and Physical Degeneration.*[3]

The study includes natives in both modernized and primitive areas: the Swiss in Switzerland; the Gaelics in the inner and outer Hebrides; the Eskimos in Alaska; Indians in the far north, west and central Canada as well as in the Western United States and Florida; the Melanesians and Polynesians on eight archipelagos in the South Pacific; tribes in central and eastern Africa; the Maori of New Zealand; plus primitive tribes in Peru and others. In spite of the differences in climate and food, or geographical locations, there was a common denominator underlying them all: food was natural, raised on good soil, and was eaten fresh and raw whenever possible.

Dr. Price is no longer living, but he has left a heritage of a nutritional road map to health. I own two copies of the book for fear something will happen to one of them and consider it worth its weight in gold for anyone who is interested in achieving and maintaining good health, as well as for prevention of illness. Why, except for the fact that he was a dentist, was Dr. Price so interested in teeth, and considered an examination of teeth and dental arches so important in this study? Most people mistakenly think of the head as an isolated part of the body and do not realize that conditions in the mouth reflect conditions in the rest of the body. Also, you can see into the mouth without assistance of X ray or exploratory surgery. The gums can tell the story of other body tissues and the teeth can indicate conditions in other bony structures in the body, as well as provide a record of the past history of the patient. A friend who became converted to good nutrition late in life visited a nutritionally-oriented dentist who observed her many filled cavities, bridges and other extensive previous dental work and said, "Well you learned the hard way!" And she had.

But even more important, Dr. Price found that tooth decay was often associated with, or was a forerunner of other body disturbances, usually degenerative diseases. He also found that I.Q.'s were higher in people with good nutrition, lower in those with poor diets. Later we will explore the tribes' basic diets in detail.

As further proof that it actually was good nutrition, not something else that was responsible for the natives' good health, no matter what tribe or geographical location, *in every case,* when civilization began to bring in such depleted food as white flour and food made from white sugar (candies and desserts other than natural fresh fruits) the state of the natives' health deteriorated![3]

What is so wrong with this civilized food? You have already witnessed the devitalization of white flour, which nowadays is further deprived of most natural nutrients, and thus becomes "empty fuel." And what is so wrong with white sugar? It, too, has been refined to the point that it contains no nutrients. For this reason it leaches the B vitamins from the body (which feed the nerves); can cause heart attacks, low blood sugar (hypoglycemia) and, of course, the well-known cavities. This fact was long ago evident to anthropologists who excavated skulls with decayed teeth in areas where "civilized foods" had been known to intrude upon native, whole, nutritious food. Dr. Price merely confirmed these facts by noting the evidence in living beings.

There are many more examples of the rape of our food which, due to lack of space, cannot be repeated here.[4] It is bad enough to have our food robbed of the healthful nutrients, and the soil overcropped or so contaminated with pesticides that it cannot support health, to say nothing of life (bugs cannot live in it). More recently the shame of additives has become a major concern.

The poor children are the main targets here. Adults are rarely mentioned in this connection but they can suffer from additives, too. There are now between *three thousand* and *five thousand* additives allowed in our foods, including artificial colors, flavors, preservatives, extenders, softeners, and many others. Some of these have been found to cause cancer. Others are a factor in allergies in both children and adults. New label laws decree that food labels are supposed to list ingredients to inform the consumer but frequently they are so hard to find, are in such small print, or in such technical terms that most buyers are unable to determine the facts. Dr. Ben Feingold discovered that these additives cause hyperactivity and unmanageability in children, who, when the additive foods are eliminated, turn into calm humans once more.

But other dangers lurk in these additive-filled foods. There are reports of headaches, asthma symptoms, and others similar to hay fever disturbances in adults as well as children. One small boy narrowly missed death, when he unsuspectingly took a bite of a food containing an allergen (for him) previously discovered by an allergist. The boy went into anaphylactic shock. Other children have taken bites of supposedly safe, common foods without reading labels and suffered throat constriction, even convulsions, in spite of warnings to avoid certain foods previously established as dangerous for that individual by an allergy specialist. The foods may sound innocent but they are not always what they seem. If you are not yet convinced that our food is being tampered with, listen to some shockers from Beatrice Trum Hunter, noted for her honesty and integrity in reporting. The following information is taken from her book, *The Great Nutrition Robbery.*[5] Here are some of the revelations she has uncovered:

> Cookies have been made experimentally with ground-up chicken feathers replacing some of the flour.
>
> Cherries used in some pies and cakes are actually calcium chloride-coated sodium alginate.
>
> Imitation cheese has been made out of banana peels, ground-up buttons, and umbrella handles.
>
> Coffee "creamers" are made of water, hydrogenated oil, sodium caseinate solids, sugar, and a host of chemical additives.
>
> Some beef cattle are fed chicken manure, sewage sludge, and ground-up wood.
>
> Ground beef is often extended by adding inferior soy protein, which absorbs up to four times its weight in water and helps to retain body fat.
>
> Sawdust (called cellulose) is often substituted for food fiber or bran in baked goods, and labelled *"natural."*

As Elizabeth Keyes says "Don't fool yourself that everything in a store is food and fit to eat."[6] No wonder so many people are ill.

WHAT CAN YOU DO?

Many people are finally wising up to what is happening to our food and you, the public, have a sword in your hands. You can refuse to buy such food. You can *read labels on everything before you buy* and boycott what you wish. I was recently surprised at a bewildered grocery store owner who discovered that some of the products on his shelf were not selling because they contained questionable additives, whereas other products, without them, sold out completely. Some customers were reading their labels which will influence his future buying. Manufacturers will sell anything to make money. They can make something good as easily as something bad if you will demand it. Write them a letter telling them why you and your friends are boycotting their products. I know it can work if enough of you will raise your voices and exert your influence. I have seen it happen.

NOTES

1. *Science*, October 3, 1946, p.312.

2. Wilfrid E. Shute, M.D., with Harald Taub, *Vitamin E for Ailing and Healthy Hearts*. New York: BJ Pub. Group, 1972.

3. Weston A. Price, D.D.S., *Nutrition and Physical Degeneration*. La Mesa, CA: Price-Pottenger Nutrition Foundation, 1945, 1970.*

4. Linda Clark, *Stay Young Longer*. New York: Pyramid Publications, 1968. Paperback edition.

5. Beatrice Trum Hunter, *The Great Nutrition Robbery*. New York: Scribners, 1978.

6. Elizabeth Keyes and Paul K. Chivington, *What's Eating You?* Marina del Rey, CA: Devorss and Co., 1978.

*Available only from the publisher. For information write: Price-Pottenger Nutrition Foundation, P.O. Box 2614, La Mesa, CA 92041.

CHAPTER THREE

Which Diet is Best for You?

Probably you are tired of hearing that you are different from everyone else in the world, but it is true and it is important to be aware of your differences. Not only are your fingerprints one of a kind, but even your blood type may vary from that of other members of your family. Also, you are influenced by your unique emotional and psychological nature, as well as your physical make-up, the latter which may show the greatest variation of all. Anatomy textbooks show innumerable pictures of various organs which vary from person to person. On an entire page of pictures of hearts in such textbooks (especially Gray's) none are the same size, the exact shape, or even located in the same place in each body. One woman, living today, was reported and photographed by a national publication as having her heart on her right side, instead of the left where it is customary. Yet she was healthy. A member of my own family, during surgical exploration, was found to have her gallbladder in a different place than expected. So, if hearts, gallbladders, kidneys and other body parts vary so widely, in shape, size, and location, it should come as no surprise that stomachs and digestive functions can also vary.

For this reason alone, it is important to realize that you may not thrive on your husband's diet, nor that of your brothers, sisters, children, or parents. Stop to think: unless you happen to be one of identical twins, triplets or quadruplets, are you or your brothers or sisters *exactly* alike in temperament and other characteristics? Your parents would be the first to say, "No," since—though you have the same parentage and environment—you are undeniably different in many ways. So you may not be able to eat like other members of your family because your needs are unique. It is cruel, if not suicidal, to demand that each child eat alike and clean up his plate or else! Of course, this does not give children license to exist on junk food, but it is only fair to cater to *important* differences in tastes, which may also indicate a need for different nutrients.

WHAT IS YOUR BASIC NATIONALITY?

To further complicate the individual problem, your ancestry may supply a clue to your food preferences as well as your needs which have become a carry-over from your genes and are still influencing you, either on an individual or a family basis. For example, if you have an Italian ancestry, you may reflect the effects of a warm climate, a longer growing season which produces abundant fruits and vegetables which may in turn cause a craving for such foods. Other Italian food favorites, such as olive oil and even pasta, are tolerated well by those with Italian ancestry, yet do not necessarily make Italians fat, but may put weight on people of other nationalities.

If your forebears were Scandinavian, you may inherit a preference for fish, an indigenous food in that area, and your genes may contain the residual need for extra minerals, present in fish. Countries rich in dairy products can produce a similar influence or need for dairy products. If you are Oriental, or have Oriental blood, an Oriental diet may suit you best, and so on.

WHERE DO YOU LIVE?

People who live in the tropics do not eat the same type of diet as those who live in Alaska. Even if you move from one area to another, your dietary needs and dietary tastes may change. Some people thrive in heat; others in cold weather. Some often lose their appetites during hot summers, so temperature can affect your dietary needs, too. Perhaps we may eventually learn that one also eats differently at different altitudes.

Add to this the great variation of individual allergies. Some people can eat cucumbers and strawberries; others dare not. So whoever coined that phrase, "One man's meat is another's poison" never spoke a truer sentence. Whatever your problem, bear in mind you are different from others and therefore must become attuned to your particular needs. The body is always trying to get well and needs your cooperation. It also does not like sudden changes. So if you wish to change your eating habits, do it gradually. Cooperate with your body; be sensitive to its wishes and its tastes as well as its needs. Don't fight it; it may be trying to tell you something!

A DOCTOR WHO DISCOVERED A DIETARY BOMB

Dr. William Donald Kelley, another D.D.S. and nutrition researcher like Dr. Weston A. Price, previously mentioned, deserves much credit because he made a discovery which proved his former theories wrong and he was brave enough to admit his mistake publicly, something that few professionals will do.

Dr. Kelley was originally convinced that everyone should be a vegetarian. He was one himself and when a patient, named Suzi, came to him with a long list of serious ailments, he not only took her case as a patient, he eventually married her! In spite of thorough medical care Suzi had been in poor health for a long time. So Dr. Kelley decided she needed some nutritional information and should become a vegetarian. Suzi acquiesced, became a vegetarian, and promptly landed in bed for an extended period, eventually lapsing into a coma for about a week. Dr. Kelley was shocked and began to reevaluate his wife's diet as well as those of his many other patients. As a result he discovered a bomb that everyone was *not* alike, could *not* eat the same diet nor even take the same vitamin/mineral supplements, *and stay well.* He began to ask his patients to let him know which foods and which supplements made them feel better or worse. He discovered that different people had different metabolisms and Suzi was no exception. She had a meat-eating metabolism, he found, and in order to be well, she needed to eat meat, especially beef, four or five times a week, a diet which he said would make *him* ill.

But Suzi recovered and is now radiantly healthy on her own type of diet, based on her unique metabolism. Other patients improved too, when they followed suit. Dr. Kelley eventually found that there are at least twelve different metabolisms and the list may have grown since then. He learned that while some people needed meat every single day, others were actually the true vegetarian types who could exist on nuts, fruits and vegetables. Still others were partial vegetarians and required some animal protein from fish, fowl or dairy products. A third type of vegetarian needed much more food than the average person, since with a poor metabolism extra food was necessary to compensate for the inability to absorb nutrients from the amount of food they had been eating.

I know two women (not Dr. Kelley's patients) who prove the fallacy that everyone can or should eat alike. One woman has been a vegetarian for fifty-five years; she thrives on it. She looks far younger than her years, can go for hours, even days with no food at all and then be satisfied with one large or several small raw salads. The other woman, approximately the same age, also looks much younger than her years, but has a completely different metabolism. She requires animal protein for energy and to avoid weakness, fatigue, anemia, even blackouts. Due to hypoglycemia, she dares not bypass a small meal or snack but must eat every few hours. I tend to be more like the second woman and can not be a vegetarian for the same reasons. So we should establish our own metabolic needs and not allow anyone to talk us out of it!

Protein is a basic need for the average person. And it is a well-known fact that vegetarians can easily develop a vitamin B_{12} deficiency. B_{12} is hard to get if one does not eat animal protein of some kind: meat, fish, fowl, or dairy products, all of which supply B_{12} liberally. B_{12} occurs very sparingly in plant foods and to get enough it is often necessary to eat pounds of such separate foods, which could also put on excess weight. Also B_{12} is hard for stomachs to assimilate in supplement form. The result of a B_{12} deficiency can be a serious nerve degeneration condition causing great weakness, fatigue and other symptoms. If these symptoms should show signs of developing, the vegetarian should run, not walk, to the nearest doctor for B_{12} injections, the speediest way to prevent nerve degeneration, which can otherwise become both chronic and fatal. Some doctors will teach the patients to administer the regular injections at home.

As you no doubt know, protein is measured by amino acid factors, of which there are many in various foods, but only eight essential ones which can be easily absorbed and used efficiently by the body. These eight essentials *must* be eaten simultaneously or else they cannot be absorbed!

Although there are twenty-two amino acids known (at this writing) the indispensable eight essential amino acids are:

1. *Methionine*—needed to help prevent convulsions, particularly during pregnancy

2. *Threonine*—a growth factor

3. *Lysine*—a lack causes irritability and fatigue. Not well distributed in vegetable proteins.

4. *Tryptophane*—an aid in capillary and blood vessel health. Recently found to be an aid for nervousness and insomnia. Also a protection against tooth decay. It can be destroyed by heat.

5. *Leucine*
6. *Isoleucine*   —both of these amino acids are growth factors.

7. *Valine*—needed for muscle stamina. A lack causes fatigue and abnormal sleepiness.

8. *Phenylanine*—another growth factor, a lack of which can cause severe mental retardation.

Information about the role of each of these amino acids is scarce, and in this case has been excerpted from various biochemical textbooks. What has been definitely established is the fact that the body cannot manufacture these amino acids, so they must be supplied in the diet. Even if one is missing from the same meal, the intake will then become an incomplete protein and cannot be used by the body successfully, even if it is added a few minutes or at a meal later on the same day. Since vegetables are usually incomplete proteins, there is danger of eventual body breakdown for most vegetarians unless animal protein or dairy products are added to the diet. Those who intelligently realize this problem and add dairy products to their diet for protection, are known as lacto-ovo-vegetarians, and are said to have a safer health future. Animal protein contains all the eight essential amino acids, and so do a few other special foods, such as brewer's yeast, which also contains most of the B vitamins as well as minerals. There are a limited number of ways out of the dilemma of bypassing animal protein for vegetarians which we will discuss shortly. Meanwhile I had not planned to repeat the list of protein needs from my other books but due to its extreme importance for your health, I am going to list the many roles protein plays in your body. It is true at first, that vegetarianism makes you feel better, since it acts as a temporary cleansing diet for the accumulation of toxins in the body, but after this point has passed, those who do not have the vegetarian metabolism and need protein, usually begin to go downhill and fast. I am reporting the value of protein because of a possible new labelling law by the government warning the public against protein foods. I want you to know the truth.

WHY IS PROTEIN SO IMPORTANT?

Prolonged deficiency of protein can cause:[1]
- anemia
- kidney disease
- liver disease
- peptic ulcer
- poor wound healing
- lack of immunity to infection
- irritability
- fatigue
- weakness
- wasting
- poor circulation
- constipation
- mental retardation in children
- edema (water storage—weight gain)
- poor vision

In addition, protein is necessary for the health and maintenance of body organs. Hormones are made of protein; so are genes, insulin, antibodies (which fight infection), secretions of the thyroid, pituitary and other glands. Even the hemoglobin or red coloring matter in the blood is made of protein!

Without protein, muscles can become weak and flabby. Muscles include not only your body and face, but your kidneys, liver, and especially your heart. All muscles are made of and are dependent on protein. Your eyes are also made of protein. Some researchers believe that the unpleasant effects of aging may be due merely to a lack of protein in those who are prone to such a deficiency. Melchior T. Dikkers, Ph.D., who researched and reported this protein list, says that the word, *protein,* of Dutch origin, means "of first importance." In other words he says, "No protein—no life!" Dr. Dikkers adds: "Research shows that all body parts (even hair and skin) need protein. No living being survives without protein."[1]

Many people become emotional about eating animal flesh. We must not forget the law of life, which is the survival of the fittest—the bigger fish eats the smaller fish, birds eat insects, all for the purpose of acquiring protein. However, if you object to this philosophy, dairy products (milk, eggs and cheese) are not the same thing as eating the animals themselves. Another alternative protein source is brewer's yeast, plus a few other complete protein foods such as soybeans (which can cause indigestion and gas for some people, and millet, to which some people, including me, are allergic).

For those who are afraid that the dairy products will cause a cholesterol problem, this has now been found to be a false conclusion. According to researcher after researcher, this has been demonstrated to be a myth.[2] Some people have eaten up to twelve eggs daily, with no rise in cholesterol! Actually your body needs cholesterol for proper functioning, particularly for the sex glands.

OTHER TIPS FOR COMPUTING PROTEIN

What about the method of combining various plants with separate amino acids to obtain all the essential factors and then eating them simultaneously for successful complete protein assimilation?

This is fine *if* you can do it; it is not easy. The healthiest vegetarian I have ever known, is a man who studied the subject in depth, as one studies any other scientific subject. Every single day he would add up his protein/amino acid content for *that* day before going to bed. If he had had too little protein he corrected the score by adding such foods as brewer's yeast before going to bed. One has to be a brain to be knowledgeable about the subject of substituting plant proteins for animal proteins. Frances Moore Lappe's book *Diet For a Small Planet* is a help here.

HOW MUCH PROTEIN IS BEST?

How much protein do you need daily? This question is answered in my books, *Secrets of Health and Beauty* and *Know Your Nutrition* and which, due to lack of space cannot be repeated here. Also remember Dr. Kelley's discovery: *What kind of a metabolism do you have?* The amount needed is also due to individual variations. Are you man or woman? Is your work physically active or sedentary? If you are a woman, are you pregnant or a nursing mother? Have you been ill long? Are you under great stress? All of these factors figure in how much protein you spend or need daily, and the more "yeses," the more protein you probably need.

CAN TOO MUCH PROTEIN BE DANGEROUS?

Of course, you recall the illnesses and deaths of some who followed the liquid protein fad diet. The explanation is an insult to Mother Nature. *NO single element* in food is isolated in Nature! Protein does not appear (grow) alone, nor do vitamins or minerals without cofactors (known as synergists) which work together to produce health. Researchers have since learned that the liquid protein diet danger was due to a lack of many accompanying minerals and some vitamins. If you tear foods apart and take out some ingredients and eat the rest, you are eating fractionated or partial food instead of the whole food. This can lead to trouble. Since the liquid protein diet did not include other nutrients or supplements on a long-term basis, many doctors agreed this was the cause of all the trouble. You also may need a special digestant for protein: HCl (hydrochloric acid). To be consistently healthy we need not one food factor here or there but *all factors,* as well as a constant variety as they occur in nature to get everything we need.

For example, Stefansson, the anthropologist, whom I knew well before his death, told me that he and a companion were trekking across the Arctic areas, when they developed excruciating headaches and thought they would die before they could reach civilization. Fortunately they met another traveler who listened to their plight, examined their knapsack of good natural foods and found the trouble: no oil. He loaned them some seal oil and the headaches vanished almost immediately. Their diet had been lopsided and seal oil was needed to balance the high protein foods, such as the jerky (dried meat) and other foods they carried with them.

Before you shudder at this oil addition, remember that Adelle Davis found that a model, who had tried every known diet to lose weight was not successful until she added about two tablespoons of the particular vegetable oil that she needed to her diet daily. So we need not *some* nutrients but *all* of them! *They all work together for health.*

The best way to obtain good nutrition is to eat whole, not fractionated, foods raised under natural conditions and on mineral rich, optimum soil without added poisons. Raw foods and unprocessed foods contain more nutrients than other foods. Even cooking interferes with some (not all) nutrients. From now on, refuse to eat foods subjected to robbery, plunder, prepared with additives, or subtracted from in any way. Read labels!

Junk foods are merely those which have *no nutritional value* but have been doctored to taste good (and sell). They merely fill you up without building up your health. They may cause "hidden hunger" which can result in weight gain. Junk foods are also usually made of white sugar and flour, stripped of all nutrients, or else, they are loaded with additives. Avoid them. Also avoid precooked foods as well as those picked green to facilitate shipping; or kept indefinitely in freezers or warehouses that have lost many nutrients. The longer the storage, the greater the loss. Substitute fresh or natural foods. One nutrition-oriented doctor, Bruce Pacetti, describes junk food as "any food that has been tampered with by man." This is undoubtedly true due to soil depletion and the fact that many of what nutrients are left are removed from the food by overprocessing. Actually, based on this definition, most of our food is reduced to junk food.

The best way to avoid junk foods is *to not buy them.* If they are not in your refrigerator or your cupboard, they can't be there to tempt you or your family. Keep on hand only wholesome foods like fresh fruits, raw vegetables, fresh nuts (preferably in the shell) and so on, which can do something for you besides just fill you up! Also, try to get your nutrition from *food,* and rely on supplements only to correct a deficiency or to fill in the gaps in your diet. Supplements mean just that: to supplement your diet, not take its place. Too many people are getting carried away and living on supplements first, and choosing food as a second fiddle.

Good food, with all nutrients present, is needed for health.

NOTES

1. Linda Clark, *Know Your Nutrition*. New Canaan, CT: Keats Publishing, Inc. 1973.
2. Richard A. Passwater, *Supernutrition for Healthy Hearts*. New York: Dial Press, 1975.

CHAPTER FOUR

Which Nutrients Are Best for You?

In these difficult times it is frustrating not to be able to find nutritionally trained doctors who can help you establish your specific type of metabolism, plus correct foods and supplements for *you*. There are several reasons for this.

Nutrition is not sufficiently taught in medical schools, so doctors are inclined to dismiss its importance and tell you just to eat a well-balanced diet and you will not need to take any vitamins or minerals. As stated before, *this is not true today*.

There are very few nutritionally trained doctors,* and those who are have had to educate themselves through reading, a method you can use, too. In fact, in many cases the public is already ahead of many orthodox doctors in nutritional knowledge. Some doctors and dietitians, wishing to attract public confidence are calling themselves nutritionists but really know little or nothing about the science. As an example, one internationally renowned nutrition researcher reports an amusing incident. Vitamins, particularly in the B vitamin family which are numerous, are labelled chronologically by numbers as well as names. The first one discovered was called Vitamin B_1, the second, B_2 and so on until the most recent discoveries of the "Bs" have now reached into the twenties.

The amusing incident reported by the well-known vitamin researcher who himself has discovered at least two new vitamins in his university laboratory, tells of the "professional" who wanted to take some B_{12} but did not have any on hand. So, the story goes, the doctor took *two vitamin B_6s instead!*

---

*For the name of a nutritional doctor in your area write to Let's LIVE Magazine, 444 North Larchmont Blvd., Los Angeles, CA 90004, enclosing a self-addressed, stamped envelope.

CORRECT FOODS RATHER THAN DRUGS

Nutritionists know that though some drugs are life savers in an emergency, they should not be used routinely since they merely mask a symptom (as an aspirin masks a headache) but do not remove the underlying cause. Correct nutrition, on the other hand, supplies deficient body elements through foods and supplements so that the body can use them to rebuild itself. But in fairness to the doctors one must admit that many patients are impatient. They demand quick relief through drugs and refuse to wait the longer interval while the body rebuilds itself more slowly through correct nutrition. As it took a long time for an ailment to develop, it takes as long for it to disappear by this natural method. Dietitians differ from nutritionists in that they prepare diets for a specific ailment, such as an ulcer, whereas a nutritionist helps the patient to supply the missing food elements for repair or to *prevent* or *reverse* the same condition.

HELPING YOURSELF

What we need today is hundreds, even thousands of doctors who use both methods, *temporarily* supplying safe drugs for pain killers (which do not produce side effects) while simultaneously providing for an intake of nutritional substances to help rebuild the body and achieve good health.

Since such doctors are not yet available in large numbers, the public is obliged to learn how to help itself. There are no schools which provide this information as we understand it, so the public needs to learn through books by reliable nutritional researchers. Remember, *you do have the right* to help yourself since it is *your* body and these books can be your guides. They have been written by such people as Adelle Davis, Drs. Emanuel Cheraskin and Carlton Fredericks, and many others—even me. All of us have devoted our lives to this research. In case you believe you cannot afford to buy books, all of them put together probably do not cost as much as the price of one day in the hospital and you will have an excellent reference library for future use.

I am finding that study groups are now pooling their interests, money and books, and studying nutrition together, with excellent results. But you will have to do your own homework and not ask health store operators to prescribe for you or even expect authors or nutritional doctors to answer questions by mail. The establishment of orthodox doctors prevents this. Nondoctors (including nutritionists) can be charged with "prescribing without a license" and severely disciplined, even jailed. So don't put any author, nutritionist or health store operator on the spot. It is a study you must pursue yourself and this is why it is important to learn how the primitive tribes studied by Dr. Price and others stayed well through what they ate.

WHAT PRIMITIVE TRIBES ATE FOR HEALTH

In general, there was no single food which proved to be a panacea. *Overall good nutrition* supplied diversified whole foods as close to their natural state as possible, and containing as many essential nutrients possible for the best state of well-being. The common denominator of all tribes, as reported by Dr. Price was, "In general, all the native foods were found to contain two to six times as high a factor of safety in the matter of body building materials as did the displacing foods" (processed foods including "foodless foods" such as white flour and white sugar brought in by civilization). All foods were eaten *whole* by the primitives, including skin, pits or seeds when possible, thus foods were not fractionated. In addition:

1. All groups studied consumed minerals and fat soluble vitamins (explained later) found in high vitamin butter, cod-liver oil, sea food or seal oil and animal organs with their fat. Dr. Price stressed quality of fats rather than quantity.

2. All foods were grown on highly mineralized soil with *no* chemical fertilizers or pesticides.

3. Many foods were eaten raw, or cooked very gently and lightly. All food was eaten in season due to problems of lack of preservation and storage. (There was no food shipping in those days.)

4. Methods of preservation and storage such as drying, freezing (in cold climates), sun-drying, and earth storage were available. Most tribes also used some form of ferments (for pickles and sauerkraut), which is a healthful shorter-term method of preservation; culturing (as in yogurt); and sprouting of seeds during non-growing seasons. Dr. Pottenger recommended fermented foods for both adults and children to improve digestion and to maintain good gastric "flora" or proper acidity.

5. Some types of sea plant or mineral, even from inland sea deposits were treasured and a part of every diet.

6. Babies were breast-fed. Children and young people were indoctrinated in good nutrition from the youngest ages to use health building foods to insure healthy future generations as well as to maintain their present health. Prenatal instruction through special protective foods was taught to young marrieds (both husband and wife) prior to bearing children. Instruction for spacing children was also given to protect the health of mothers as well as their offspring.

7. Exercise and games were encouraged for all ages. Pure air and sunlight were taken for granted as necessary for everyone.

8. Sweets, except fruits, were rarely used.

9. In each tribe, the daily diet contained some types of raw, unaltered protein: sprouted seeds, milk, eggs, nuts, sea foods and meats.

Although meat was not plentiful nor eaten often, other forms of protein were. Dr. Price said, "As yet I have not found a single group of primitive racial stock which was building and maintaining excellent bodies by living entirely on plant foods (vegetarianism)." The photographs in Dr. Price's book show that the natives, both men and women, on such optimum diets were far better looking—the women, more beautiful, the men more handsome, than those who were existing on refined or inadequate foods.

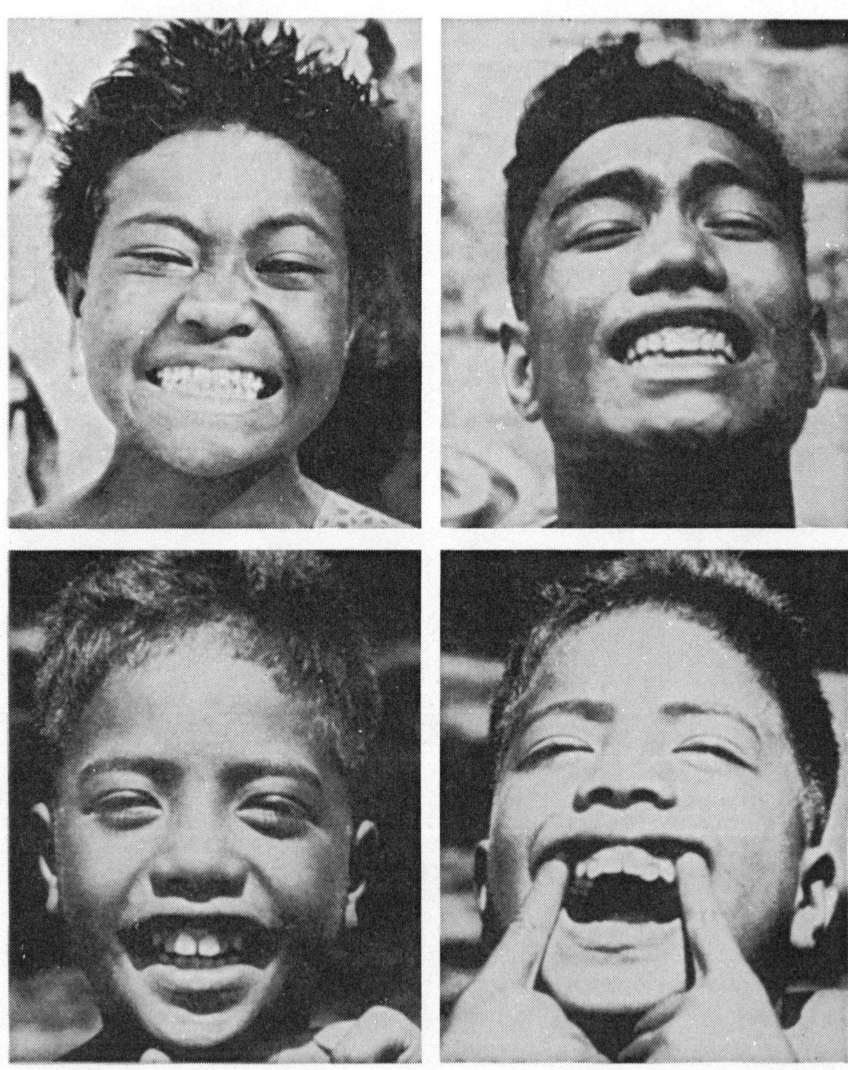

Note the marked difference in facial and dental arch form of the two adult Samoans above and the two youngsters below. The facial bones are underdeveloped, causing a marked constriction of the arches with crowding of the teeth. This is a typical expression of inadequate nutrition of the parents.

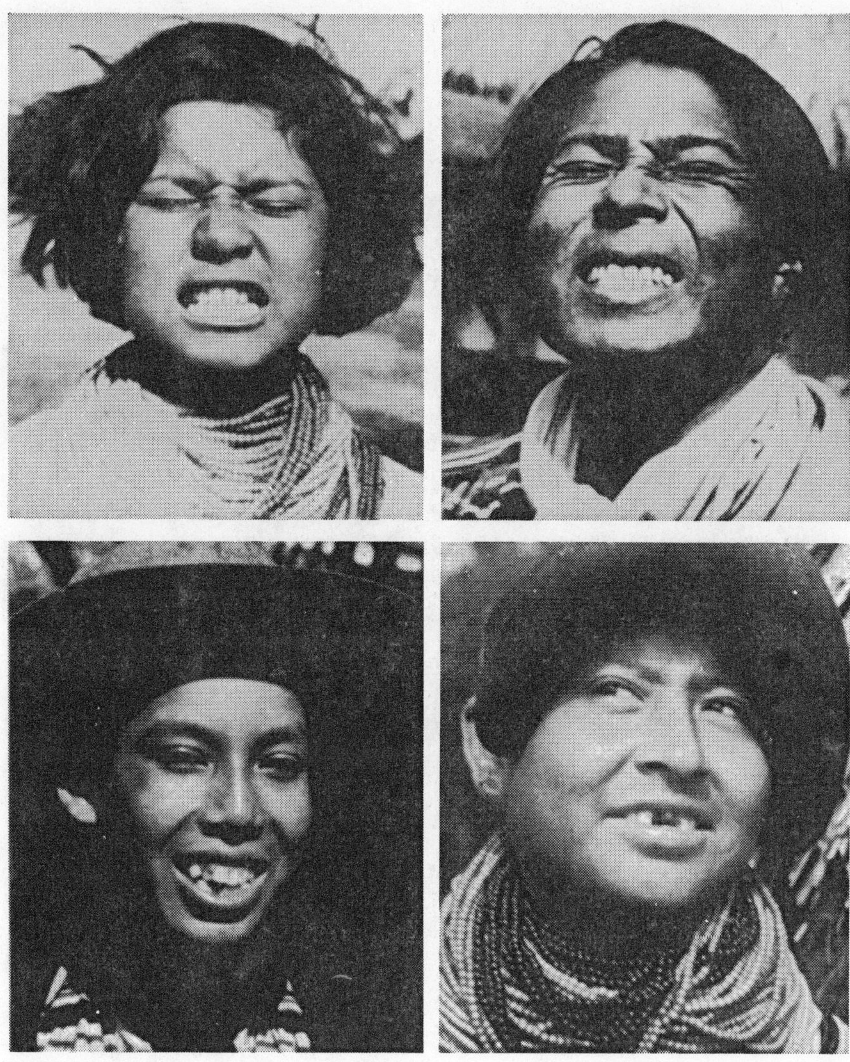

Here again, the contrast between the natives on primitive diets and those on modernized diets is striking. Note the change in these Seminole Indians in Florida. The lower photos depict the marked lack of development of the facial bones with a narrowing of the nostrils and dental arches. Their faces are stamped with the blight which so many think of as normal because it is so common with us.

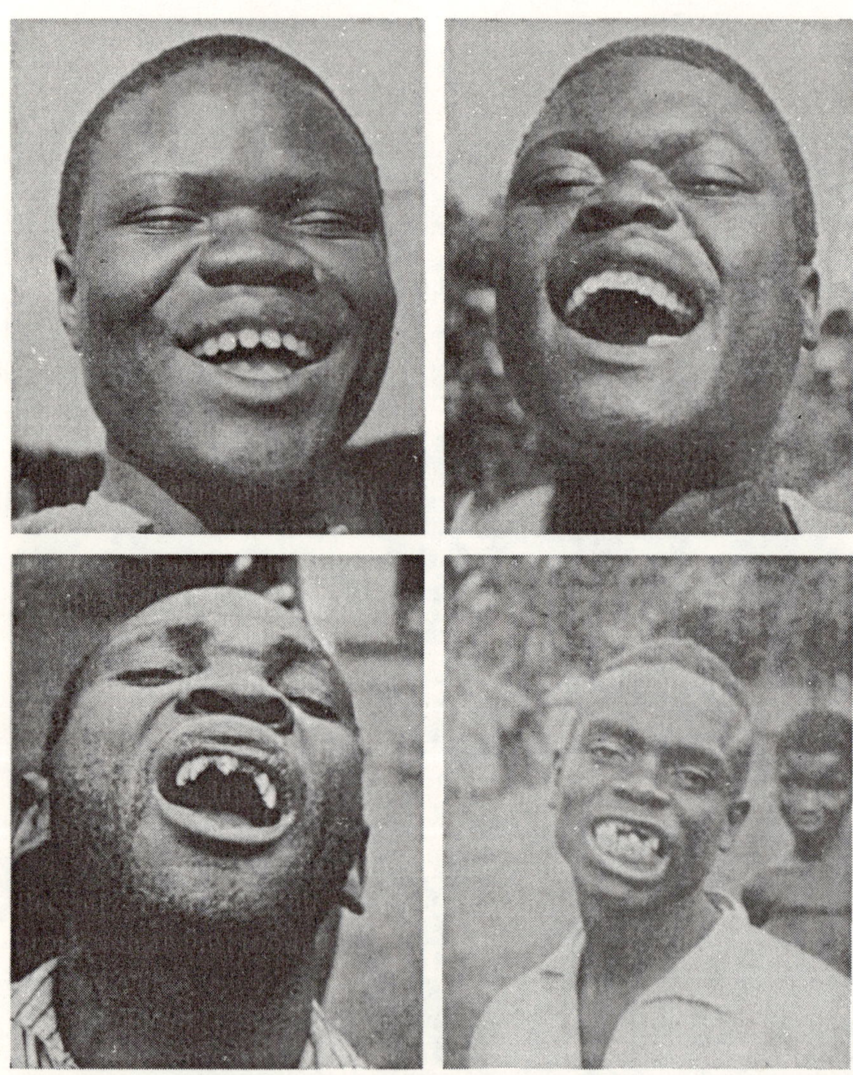

The reward of obeying nature's laws of nutrition is illustrated here. Note the breadth of the dental arches and the finely proportioned features above. Their bodies are as well-built as their heads. The Africans below have adopted the foods of modern commerce. The cases shown here are typical of workers on plantations which use imported foods. Even their magnificent heredity could not protect them.

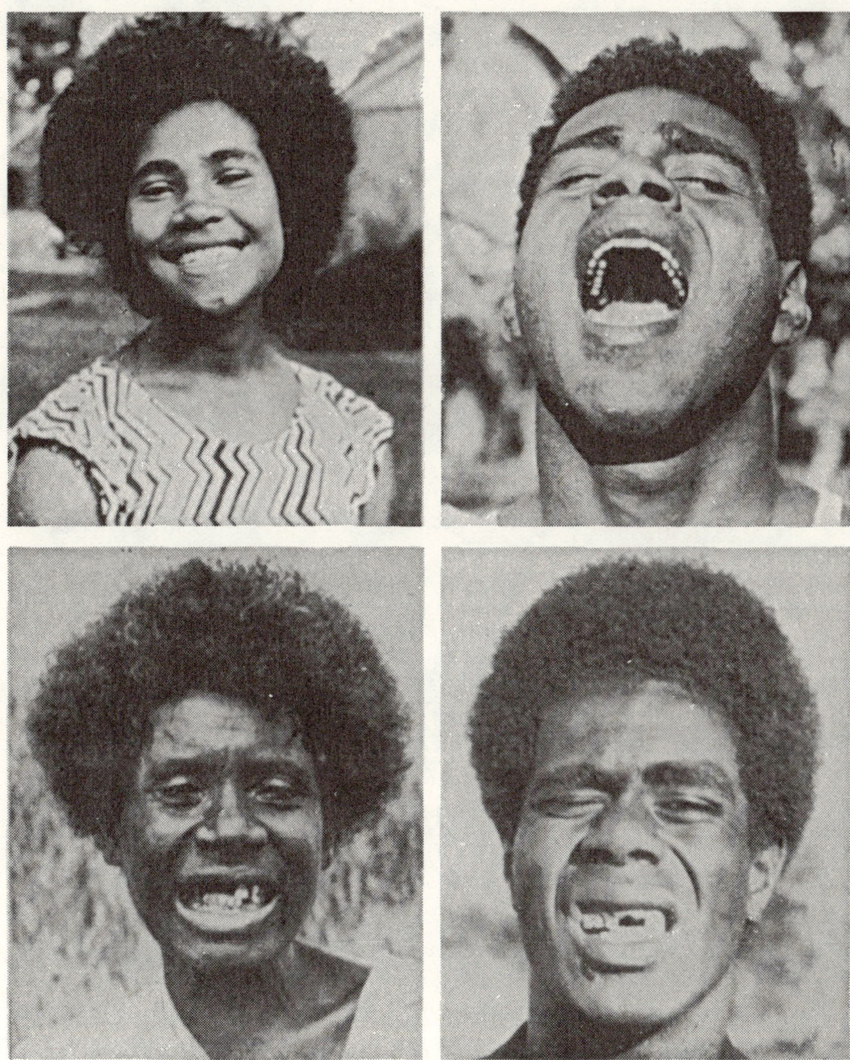

The development of the facial bones determines the size and shape of the palate and the size of the nasal air passages. Note the strength of the neck of the man above and the well proportioned face of the girl. The photographs below illustrate the effect of changing from the native food to the imported foods of commerce.

MAJOR FOODS EATEN BY VARIOUS TRIBES

Swiss of the Loetschental Valley:
- whole rye bread
- dairy products
- meat once weekly due to shortages
- vegetables, fresh in summer, stored in winters

Tribes in the Outer Hebrides:
- oatmeal
- fish, including cod-livers and heads

Eskimos:
- fish, dried or frozen
- animal organs and tissues (more nutritious than muscle meats)
- a few berries, including cranberries (a source of vitamin C)
- fish eggs (a source of vitamin E)
- seal oil

Indians of Northern Canada:
- wild game: moose and caribou, with emphasis on organ meats (muscle meats were fed to the dogs)
- bone marrow, and bones cut fine, as close to modern bone meal as possible
- summers—growing plants
- winters—tree buds and bark

South Pacific and Australian Tribes:
- shell fish and scale fish
- plant roots, fruits, raw and cooked, taro and poi, (both fermented)
- young leaves for greens
- coconut cream made from hand-ground coconut meal, and water, and baked in green leaves

African Natives:
- sweet potatoes
- beans, cereals
- some cereals, including millet and corn

> • large quantities of fish
> • animal meat, both wild and domesticated

Aborigines of Australia:
> • wild plants and animals, with emphasis on organs
> • sea foods

Maoris of New Zealand:
> • sea food in abundance. some birds
> • green plants, roots, fruits

Dr. Price observed excellent teeth in New Zealand children and asked their schoolteachers what the children brought from home in their lunches. The teachers said they brought nothing but when school was dismissed at midday, the children rushed to the beach, built fires, dived after lobsters and roasted and ate them on the spot.

Indians of Peru:
> • native animals, including guinea pigs
> • fish eggs, fresh or dried (claimed by the natives to provide fertility for women)
> • dried kelp (seaweed) to prevent "big neck" or goiter (kelp is rich in iodine)
> • potatoes

This partial list is merely a condensation of the general type of natural food favored by assorted tribes, and which varied according to the indigenous foods found or grown in their areas. Obviously, being natural, fresh and whole, they were all highly nutritious, with an abundance of minerals, some fat soluble vitamins, etc., vitamin C and enzymes (in raw foods), all derived from their *natural* food, raised on *natural* soil or in *natural* waters. Today we know that there are two classifications of vitamins—the water soluble and the fat or oil soluble. The fat soluble vitamins A, D, E, F, and K, *require* some fat in the diet in order to be properly assimilated.

In addition to the fat soluble vitamins, there are the water soluble ones, which are not stored in the body as are the fat soluble vitamins. These include all of the B family (a big one) plus vitamin C. Water solubles can be washed out of the body by excess beverages, alcohol, coffee, tea, even diuretics. Sugar and alcohol also leach B vitamins out of the body: the B vitamins basically contribute to the health of the nervous system. (For further information on the roles each vitamin plays, see my book, *Know Your Nutrition,* in paperback at health stores).

NATURAL VERSUS SYNTHETIC VITAMINS

Unfortunately today we do not have the optimum food conditions as those enjoyed by primitive tribes. For example, our soils are over-cropped, causing in many cases nutritionally depleted plants. As proof, several years ago Dr. Firman E. Bear of the Department of Agricultural Chemistry, Rutgers University, analyzed 204 samples of vegetables grown in the same season and at the same stage of growth. Dr. Bear examined the plants with the help of a radar-type machine. Two carrots could look alike to the naked eye, but the sensitive machine established that one carrot could be highly nutritious whereas another was nutritionally worthless. Different soil conditions were found to be responsible: depleted soils produced depleted plants or vegetables. This means that when you go to a store, you have no way of knowing which vegetable is high or low in nutrition. The only solution is to know your farmer and his practices in raising food, or grow your own.

Since our food today is nutritionally questionable this explains why it may be necessary to fill in the gaps of our diet with vitamin/mineral supplements. Obviously we would prefer those which are natural to synthetics, but here we run into an obstacle. Scientists and chemists claim that there is absolutely no difference between synthetic and natural supplements. In fact some manufacturers insist that there is no such thing as a natural supplement.

Fortunately, there is another side to this story. It is no doubt true that a synthetic vitamin may be identical, molecule for molecule, to a *fractionated* or separate vitamin. *But Nature does not grow such vitamins.* In natural plants and other nutrient sources, vitamins do not appear singly but in combination with other cofactors, called synergists, which help those vitamins to be assimilated by the body! The synthetic vitamins, on the other hand, appear in single form

VARIATIONS in MINERAL CONTENT in VEGETABLES. (Firman E. Bear report. Rutgers Uni.)

	Percentage of dry weight		Millequivalents per 100 grams dry weight				Trace Elements parts per million dry matter				
	Total Ash or Mineral Matter	Phosphorus	Calcium	Magnesium	Potassium	Sodium	Boron	Manganese			Cobalt
SNAP BEANS											
Highest	10.45	0.36	40.5	60.0	99.7	8.6	73	60	227	69	0.26
Lowest	4.04	0.22	15.5	14.8	29.1	0.0	10	2	10	3	0.00
CABBAGE											
Highest	10.38	0.38	60.0	43.6	148.3	20.4	42	13	94	48	0.15
Lowest	6.12	0.18	17.5	15.6	53.7	0.8	7	2	20	0.4	0.00
LETTUCE											
Highest	24.48	0.43	71.0	49.3	176.5	12.2	37	169	516	60	0.19
Lowest	7.01	0.22	16.0	13.1	53.7	0.0	6	1	9	3	0.00
TOMATOES											
Highest	14.20	0.35	23.0	59.2	148.3	6.5	36	68	1938	53	0.63
Lowest	6.07	0.16	4.5	4.5	58.8	0.0	5	1	1	0	0.00
SPINACH											
Highest	28.56	0.52	96.0	203.9	257.0	69.5	88	117	1584	32	0.25
Lowest	12.38	0.27	47.5	46.9	84.6	0.8	12	1	19	0.5	0.00

only, without the cofactors or synergists. And tests show that those who take these nutrients in natural form usually get better results in the long run than from taking synthetics. So the synthetics supply you with isolated factors only, instead of the full complex or combination of the nutrient plus the cofactors which it has grown. This can make a lot of difference.

Cod-liver oil is an example. Doctors and others have prescribed it for rickets (a calcium deficiency disturbance) for many years with success. We know that cod-liver oil contains vitamins A, D, F and others. Yet these same vitamins given separately in synthetic form do not seem, even to doctors, as successful in combating rickets as cod-liver oil, a whole natural product with many nutrients present (some investigators claim there are sixty nutrients in it). The natural vitamins A, D, and F and possibly others in cod-liver oil, are known to help the body assimilate calcium so greatly needed in cases of rickets. The average orthodox doctor will agree, and usually prefer the whole natural food product to the separate synthetic supplements. On the other hand, in some cases a synthetic vitamin *may* be successful if used alone. Ascorbic acid, one factor of the whole vitamin C family, is a synthetic which seems to work alone successfully in some situations.

One manufacturer of so-called natural supplements, who is no longer living, admitted to me that his company added synthetic, isolated B vitamins to a base of liver or brewer's yeast, each a whole natural product, and labelled the final formula: *Natural.*

Some people, without realizing it, are accomplishing the same results. They take a synthetic vitamin (since it seems to be the only thing they can find) and add the whole food from which it came containing the vitamin *and* its synergists.

This is effective since all factors missing from the separate synthetics are thus supplied.

HOW TO COMPENSATE FOR NUTRIENT LOSS

Adelle Davis wrote in her book, *Let's Eat Right to Keep Fit,* ''Let us be cautious in feeling secure that a mere capsule of mixed B vitamins will supply the missing requirements . . . [instead] our needs must be met largely by wholesome foods chosen with the utmost care.''

This advice, then, gives us the clue to health also discovered by Dr. Price's primitive tribes: get *all* nutrients in your diet from whole, not partial food, raised naturally on whole, natural soil, uncontaminated by pesticides. *Do not try to live on supplements alone* but do use every type of whole, natural food possible. Add supplements only as insurance against a deficiency of nutrients you may suspect in yourself or your food.

Very recently a few real natural supplements have begun to appear on the market. These supplements are made from whole foods, with nothing added, nothing removed. Read your labels to identify them. We hope more will follow. This method of fortifying your diet can also apply to your cooking. If you are using a traditional recipe, say for biscuits made with unbleached white flour (which is minus the wheat germ) add some wheat germ to the recipe or take some vitamin E separately.

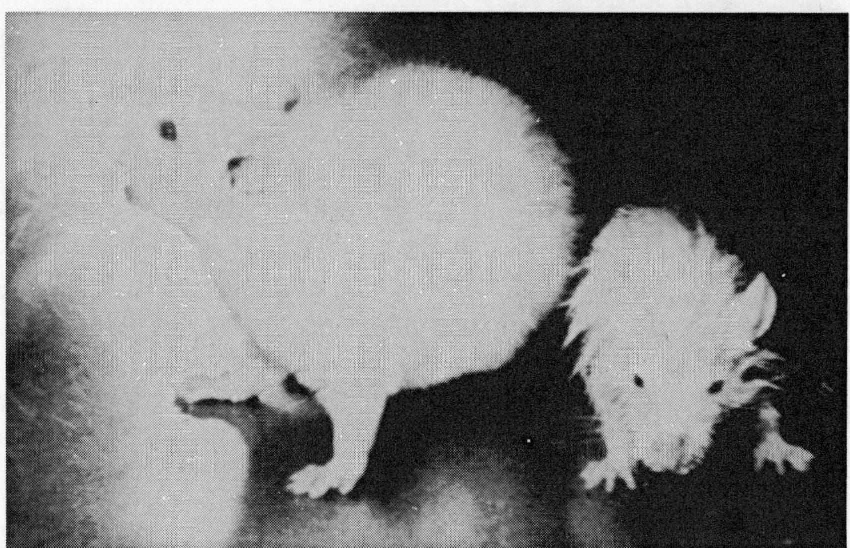

Natural versus Artificial Food. Weanling rats fed shell eggs (left) and commercial *Eggbeaters* (right). Based on the original formula of *Eggbeaters*.

Reprinted by permission of the author, F. A. Kummero, Ph.D., Burnside Research Laboratory, University of Illinois, Champaign, IL 60801, and the journal *Pediatrics*, 53(4): 565-570, copyright American Academy of Pediatrics 1974.

Orientals who use polished white rice, from which the coating, which contains the entire B vitamin family is removed, make up for this loss, perhaps intuitively, by using soy sauce and other foods which include B vitamins. In fact one of the new, all natural supplements just appearing, is a B complex product made from whole rice with the B vitamin rich coating.

HIGH POWER FOODS

These foods, sometimes called "wonder foods" merely contain more nutrients than the average foods and laboratory analyses prove it.[1] Blackstrap molasses, wheat germ, brewer's yeast, raw sunflower seeds, yogurt and others provide you with a rich source of nutrients plus their synergists, all in a single food. Even whole brown rice could qualify as a power food. Why buy white rice only to have to buy separately B vitamins removed from brown rice as an expensive supplement? Brown rice contains the whole B vitamin family and their synergists and is delicious. It is a bit nuttier and less mushy than white rice. I serve brown rice exclusively. Although there is a slight difference in appearance, texture and flavor, most people consider it more delicious.

There are nutritional cookbooks available at health stores to help you cook these "new" foods. Ask to see the ones by Adelle Davis, Agnes Toms, Beatrice Trum Hunter, the Price-Pottenger Nutrition Foundation's *Guide to Living Foods* and others. Don't go overboard all at once and alienate your family to these good foods. Try a few now and then until you find those which are popular. Don't push too hard or they will resist your efforts. Some of my most successful recipes I found in these special cookbooks. They include a tamale pie, popovers, a great French green salad and Thanksgiving turkey which is always a success. You can find your own.

In summary, keep the following in mind:

As stated in *Natural Health World* (a monthly publication, March 1979), "Stay away from food that goes through a factory before it gets to you. In factories, the good parts of food are taken out by refining, and the bad stuff, like preservatives, nitrates, nitrites, artificial flavorings and other additives are put in. In other words, eat natural food as much as possible."

And don't blame our contamined air and water for everything. Dr. D. T. Quigley, of Omaha, Nebraska, an M.D. who did research similar to that of Dr. Price, wrote, "In the life of the ordinary person the most common disease-producing factors are from food deficiencies. While contaminated air and water can occasionally produce disease, it is not to be compared in importance with the amount of disease produced by errors in [incomplete] diet." (from *Acres U.S.A.*, March 1979)

So the message from those who know is the same: *Eat Naturally!*

NOTES

1. Linda Clark, *Know Your Nutrition*. New Canaan, CT: Keats Publishing, Inc., 1973.

CHAPTER FIVE

Don't Shortchange Minerals!

Although minerals have been known far longer than vitamins, the excitement of the discovery of vitamins in the early 1900's seemed to eclipse minerals. Yet minerals are considered far more important than vitamins! Dr. Charles Northen, M.D., one of the earliest nutritional physicians, said, "It is not commonly realized that the vitamins control the body's appropriation of minerals, *but in the absence of minerals, vitamins have no function*. Lacking vitamins, the system can make use of the minerals, but lacking minerals, the vitamins are useless."[1]

Dr. Price, on his return home following his study of the primitive tribes, analyzed in his laboratory samples of foods consumed by those he found to be healthy. The analyses revealed that the foods eaten by them contained from four up to seventy-five times more than the amount of minerals in foods consumed by less healthy natives. These mineral-rich foods came from sea foods—sea plants and fish—plus land plants grown on naturally mineralized soil.[2]

Another remote tribe, sometimes called the Healthy Hunzas, who live in the Himalayas, have been studied by visitors and researchers to determine why this tribe is so healthy, happy, free from all disease, including cancer, and enjoy unusual longevity. (Doctors are not only *not* needed but do not even exist in this country.) Various theories have been advanced, such as the complete freedom from pollution of air, water and soil. Some visitors have seized upon their own particular pet theory, such as assuming that little or no meat, or fat, or processed foods is the explanation. The general consensus, however, is that the water, which cascades down over the mountains is loaded with minerals. When the water is poured into a drinking glass, the silt settles at the bottom of the glass, while the natives drink the cloudy water above it.

A story was told by a doctor who many years ago attended the delivery of a baby boy who was extremely puny at birth. In desperation, the doctor took the child home and tried every type of food, none of which stayed down. Finally he tried the various minerals in homeopathic form called cell salts, about which he had just learned. He made a solution of these cell salts and fed them to the baby by eyedropper. They not only stayed down, they saved the child's life. For three years the boy had no solid food of any kind but lived exclusively on all twelve of the cell salts (each representing a different mineral). Eventually, the doctor adopted the child and after he grew to manhood and entered the military service, the army doctors were overwhelmed at the young man's excellent physical condition.[3]

Minerals play many roles. Some researchers have conjectured that aging may actually be due to a cumulative deficiency of minerals in the body.

Types of Minerals

There are three general types of minerals: Major, minor and toxic.

The major or essential minerals occur in larger amounts in the body, and thus are needed in greater amounts. The minor minerals are no less important; they merely occur in tiny amounts and are called trace minerals or micronutrients. The toxic minerals are known as the heavy metals and are troublemakers, so obviously should be avoided; or if already present in the body, should be eliminated.

CALCIUM

Calcium is found in the body not only in the bony structure (this includes teeth) but also in the extracellular fluids and soft tissues as well. Bone is constantly being reformed and absorbed, so an intake of calcium is continuously needed to meet these constantly changing requirements. Otherwise, one part of the body will borrow from another part, on the principle of "robbing Peter to pay Paul" leaving a deficiency or debt somewhere in the body to be repaid. This is particularly true of teeth which may develop cavities not only from an attack by local factors such as sugary foods, but because the bony structure can be undermined and weakened by a general body calcium deficiency. A calcium deficiency can also lead to osteoporosis (bone loss), inadequate blood clotting, excitable nerves, brittle fingernails, muscle cramps and insomnia.

Calcium may be liberally taken into the body by milk and dairy foods but may not necessarily be assimilated. Acid in the form of vitamin C, HCl or diluted apple cider vinegar is often used to dissolve calcium so that it will not pile up in the joints as arthritis, and protein is needed for better calcium metabolism, too. Vitamin D (from sunshine or supplement form) is a *must* for calcium absorption, though many studies warn that *no more than 400 units daily in supplement form should be used.* Since Vitamin D is one of the oil soluble vitamins, it can be stored in the body and excesses have been found dangerous. The minimum recommendation of *calcium* per adult daily is about 800 mgs. This is because tests show that 320 mgs. of calcium are lost daily by an adult and only 40% of dietary calcium is absorbed. The 800 mgs. provide sufficient coverage to allow for loss and to establish calcium equilibrium in the body in the average person.[4]

PHOSPHORUS

Phosphorus is really no real problem. Since it occurs in nearly all foods, a deficiency is unusual. Not only that, but some of the B vitamins need to be combined with dietary phosphorus in order to be effective.

There are only two problems to watch for in connection with phosphorus. The mineral acts almost like a twin to calcium. They attach themselves to each other thus can be excreted from the body simultaneously. This could lead (and has led) to a calcium deficiency. For example, if you are taking large amounts of lecithin, (an important substance, high in phosphorus) watch out for muscle cramps, a sign of calcium deficiency. Either lower the amount of lecithin (phosphorus) or increase the intake of calcium to correct the imbalance. Many a person has taken calcium tablets to successfully outwit muscle cramps.

A second problem with phosphorus is that a deficiency can be caused by taking antacids! The resulting symptoms are weakness, lack of appetite, fatigue and pain in the bones. The situation is easily corrected by merely stopping the antacids![5]

MAGNESIUM

Magnesium is a relatively new mineral discovery, and a bell ringer. Its lack has been found to cause extreme nervousness, hair loss, muscular excitability, tremors, neuromuscular disorders, convulsions, even epilepsy, as well as disturbances in heart and kidney function, plus hormone imbalances. It has led to kidney stones and the "shakes" in an alcoholic and spasms in drug addicts, as well as ulcers and infections in others. Magnesium activates over 5,000 different body enzyme reactions, is involved in protein synthesis, vitamin utilization and muscle contraction. It is an extremely important mineral. It is usually taken with calcium.

IRON

Iron is a familiar mineral to most people who connect anemia and fatigue with its lack. OK, but there is more to it than that. Beware of overloading on inorganic iron, which can destroy vitamin E in the stomach. *Inorganic* iron and vitamin E should be taken eight to twelve hours apart. This is not a problem with natural or organic iron. There are many types of anemia or even fatigue, and lack of iron is not the only cause. Anemia can also result from a deficiency of vitamin B_{12}, or even vitamin E. If you must take an iron supplement be sure it is taken from a dietary source, such as liver.

Many nutritionists are worried about the elimination of iron, among other natural substances, in cereals and flours, and the addition of synthetic substances, including synthetic iron—all products termed "enriched." This, like the history of vitamin E, is another robbery of nature's bounty. In "enriched foods" many nutrients are robbed from a natural food and only a few synthetics are restored, a pure case again of fractionated food. Actually, iron is kind of a crazy mineral. The more you take, the less is absorbed, and the less you have, the better the absorption.

Iron, like calcium, definitely needs acid for its assimilation. This could also be in the form of HCl, (taken as a supplement if your own is waning), or vitamin C, or if all else is unavailable, diluted apple cider vinegar. It is true, that due to menstruation, women are more susceptible to iron deficiency than men, but if this is the case, again lean on natural dietary sources, such as liver if possible, fresh or desiccated, rather than a synthetic chemical, which has caused trouble for many. This is one case when, if you eat a diet rich in natural nutrients, including those found in animal and dairy proteins, whole grains and other whole foods, and make sure your acid content is also sufficient to help your body utilize the natural iron, you should be OK. If you are still weak, wan and pale, there is another natural iron supplement available at health stores called *Hemolasses.*

Ferrum Phos. (Iron Phosphate), is a homeopathic cell salt and an easily assimilated form of iron, available from homeopathic pharmacies. Cell salts come in little sweet pellets which are usually not swallowed with water, but allowed to dissolve on or under the tongue in order to be absorbed by osmosis into the tissues. Blackstrap molasses is another natural source of iron, but after taking it from the spoon, be sure to rinse your mouth. It can erode tooth enamel.

Iron deficiency is common among vegetarians since most vegetables contain little iron. Some vegetarians have had to resort to taking liver (which they call their "medicine") or injections of B_{12}, to correct the deficiency symptoms from lack of iron.

COPPER

Watch out for copper. It is a trace mineral and a cofactor which naturally cooperates with iron, but so many plumbing pipes are now made of copper that there is rarely a lack of it. Actually, in many cases excessive copper can cause toxic levels to appear. The best way to avoid this is to let your water run for a few seconds in the morning before using, if it has remained in the copper pipes overnight.

MANGANESE

Manganese is another comparative newcomer. It helps chromium to assist in fat and carbohydrate assimilation as well as help control glucose tolerance. Its lack can cause dizziness, loss of coordination, paralysis and convulsions. Manganese is also a muscle mineral. If you have had a chiropractic or osteopathic adjustment and want it to stay in place longer, take manganese! It has worked for me.

ZINC

Zinc is a newcomer and we are having a hard time keeping up with the new benefits constantly being discovered. It is definitely a "good guy."

Zinc can help a poor appetite, improve your senses of taste and smell or help them return if lost. It has helped prostate trouble in men, and it is also used to stop body odor, help arthritis and accelerate wound healing. It has also slowed or stopped hair loss.

From 15 to 30 mgs. are recommended for daily use. On chelated labels (a method to help assimilation) read the *elemental* amount present for the correct dosage. Zinc in the diet is found in meat, fish, whole grains, liver, eggs, and seeds such as pumpkin and sunflower seeds. A recent survey in *The National Enquirer* (April 17, 1979) stated that zinc has caused a dramatic improvement in millions of people, and this publication called it "a magic mineral."

SODIUM AND POTASSIUM

These two minerals are like two horses which separately pull in opposite directions, but pulling together in the same direction can insure smoother progress. Working together as a team they produce what is known as the sodium-potassium ratio balance.

Sodium helps to store water in the body; potassium releases it. There is such a delicate balance involved in order to prevent a deficiency of either mineral that a driver is needed to coordinate them. This driver is vitamin B_6 which, when taken in supplemental form protects the delicate sodium-potassium ratio. Too much or too little of either of these minerals has caused trouble, but B_6 acts as a safeguard, as researched by John M. Ellis, M.D., who describes in his book how premenstrual irritability in women and smaller waistlines in men were achieved by no other means than the use of vitamin B_6.[6] It is also used for nausea in pregnancy.

IODINE

Iodine (a trace mineral) is involved with the thyroid in producing energy. Like many other minerals, you can overdo iodine, so rather than take it as a separate supplement, it is safer to take food which contains it. Iodine is found in sea plants, usually kelp, as well as in fish. Most land vegetables are low in iodine.

I have been told, but cannot prove, that government food regulations have tried—and perhaps succeeded in removing iodine from kelp, an otherwise excellent source of all minerals. If this is true, what a pity! Some nutritionists believe the only safe way to take iodine is by using iodized salt. A lack of iodine in geographical areas where iodine is deficient in the soil has been established as a cause of goiter.

Broda O. Barnes, M.D., goes still further. He supplies some impressive research that hypo-thyroidism (low thyroid function) may not only be accompanied by low energy but his findings show that this disturbance may also be *the* major cause of heart attacks. Instead of using iodine as a corrective, he uses (by prescription only) a natural source of the thyroid hormone. I have witnessed a "coming-alive" of people who have used this therapy. Dr. Barnes tells in his book how to find out for yourself at home if your thyroid function is low, making you a candidate for these disturbances.[7] Those whose thyroid is normal, instead of using the natural thyroid substance, usually depend upon the iodine in kelp and other sea plants to prevent thyroid malfunction as well as to keep their energy level high.

SELENIUM

Selenium, another trace mineral, seems to be a two-edged sword. It is considered to be a cofactor of Vitamin E, to be useful in preventing cancer and birth defects. This may possibly be true, but there is another side of the story. As a trace mineral the safe recommended dose is only *50 micrograms per person, per day,* a very tiny amount. Selenium, then, may pose a hazard for those who believe that if a little is good, more is better. To complicate the situation selenium occurs in the soils only in certain areas.

According to W. D. Currier, M.D. (*Let's LIVE* June 1979), high-selenium states in the U.S. which contain in some cases as much as three hundred percent higher amounts than is found in selenium-poor states, include Texas, Oklahoma, Arizona, Colorado, Louisiana, Utah, Alabama, Nebraska, Kansas, North and South Dakota. The low selenium states are: Connecticut, Illinois, Ohio, Oregon, Massachusetts, Rhode Island, New York, Pennsylvania, Indiana and Delaware.

If, and I do mean *if,* you are living in one of these areas where soil selenium is high and you are eating foods raised there, be careful. If you are also taking selenium supplements (it is available not only separately but in some specially prepared brewer's yeast tablets, each tablet containing the recommended 50 micrograms) watch it! A recent news release reported the mysterious death of several farmers who were found dead in one of the Dakota states, a high selenium soil area. The cause of the deaths according to this report: too much selenium. It may be safer to get this mineral which is balanced correctly with other minerals in your diet. It occurs in broccoli, wheat germ, whole grains, and garlic. I would say play it safe. According to Dr. Carl C. Pfeiffer, too much selenium can cause such toxic effects as loss of hair, nails, teeth, and progressive paralysis.[8]

Dr. Robert M. Downs and Jack J. Challem, in an article, "A Primer of Minerals" (*Let's LIVE* March 1979) state, "Selenium poses paradoxes. It is essential in trace quantities, yet in larger amounts it can be one of the most dangerous substances known to man."

Chromium

Chromium, another trace mineral, may have a brilliant future. It has been found to consistently, though gradually, improve glucose tolerance. This means new help for diabetics. In fact, one enthusiastic chromium researcher told me that he believed, through the correct use of chromium, that diabetes may possibly disappear within the next fifteen years. He advises a very small amount, no higher than .2 mgs. or 200 micrograms daily, of the elemental form of chromium (see your labels).

Other trace minerals are molybdenum, nickel, tin, vanadium, silicon, cobalt (a constituent of B_{12}) and others. Although there is some knowledge available about these newer trace elements, the search is not yet complete.

THE TOXIC MINERALS

So far, we have discussed the minerals which, if used with a little common sense, can be classified as "good guys." Not so with the following which are known as the "bad guys." Avoid them like the plague! They are also known as the heavy metals: lead, cadmium, mercury; and possibly if not probably, especially if taken alone, aluminum and arsenic.

I will tell you the danger, the symptoms, as well as the antidote of each of the heavy metals. Minerals are a fascinating subject and entire books have been written about them, but lack of space prevents repeating all information here. If you wish still more help, there is a small easy-to-read booklet which sells for only one dollar and is available from Health Evaluations, Inc., P.O. Box 187, Hayward, California, 94543. I have included much of the documented information in the following discussion of the toxic metals from this source, but the book also discussed the good, essential minerals. It is one of the most informative as well as inexpensive sources of mineral knowledge I have found. This organization which prepared and published it is a nonprofit group. Simply ask for the mineral information book, enclosing the small fee—a real value. It should answer most of your questions.

Now for those "bad guys" the toxic metals, which include lead, mercury and cadmium, and perhaps aluminum and arsenic.

LEAD

Some	muscle weakness
symptoms	tremors
of lead	gout
poisoning:	lack of coordination, clumsiness symptoms similar to multiple sclerosis.

One woman, whose symptoms of great fatigue and even blackouts, defied all doctors who examined her. They told her it was her imagination. Hair tests finally revealed a high lead residue, which was traced to drinking coffee from a pewter cup which contained lead.

Other sources of lead:
- auto exhaust, smog and other environmental sources
- soft water in lead plumbing (let water run in the morning before using)
- some hair colorings
- lead paints
- some ceramic glazes

Antidote:
Calcium
Vitamin C
Baked beans (contains a lead antagonist, glutathione, as found by J. J. Miller, Ph.D.).[1] Also, from *Textbook of Biochemistry* Harrow-Mazur, Seventh Edition

MERCURY

Symptoms:	fatigue
	headaches and forgetfulness
	convulsions
	kidney damage
	numbness or tingling of fingers and mouth; difficult enunciation
	dimming of vision

Sources: —large fish such as swordfish and tuna (if eaten
                      regularly)
                    —pesticides, fungicides, chemical fertilizers
                    —dental amalgams
                    —calomel
                    —fluorescent lights (if mercury vapor type)
                    —many others

Antidote:
   garlic
   apple sauce, another Dr. Miller discovery, possibly explained by
   pectin, a poison neutralizer.[1]
   Hepar Sulph 6x potency, a homeopathic remedy from homeopathic pharmacies listed in my book.[1]

CADMIUM

Symptoms: high blood pressure
                    atherosclerosis and possible heart attack
                    stroke

Sources: —tap water from galvanized or plastic plumbing
                      pipes (let run after standing overnight)
                    —refined foods, processed meats
                    —cigarette smoke
                    —cola drinks
                    —instant coffee

Antidote:
   Zinc

For some people, copper is a poison. Zinc plus manganese are anti-
dotes (Pfeiffer). Aluminum and arsenic are also questionable as
poisoners. Arsenic has been used to spray strawberries in fields by
helicopters. I have seen them! Arsenic is also used to spray chicken
houses, eventually contaminating chicken livers which are the poison
filters for animals as well as people. It is true that arsenic is used in

small amounts as a medicine, yet many believe it is cumulative in the body, the toxicity finally becoming fatal. Used in balanced amounts in a natural multimineral product, it is apparently safe.

I view aluminum with distrust after being told by a responsible doctor that in Europe many cases of arthritis are traceable to aluminum. Aluminum poisoning is possible and many people have eliminated their aluminum cooking ware for this reason.

Both vitamins C and E are believed to be helpful in eliminating the heavy metals. Nutritionists also believe that if you are saturated with all the good essential minerals, you will resist the entrance of much of the heavy metals into your system.

Combined minerals, taken in natural form simultaneously are usually in balance, thus safe. They are found in kelp, and other combinations such as Minerals 72 and Azomite (see pages 150-151) available in health stores. They are also available individually, with the exception of some of the newer ones which can be added separately, in cell salt form (like the ones the doctor gave to the baby) and sold in homeopathic pharmacies. Homeopathic minerals are also available in combination form.

HOW TO TEST FOR HEAVY METALS

The most common method at present of locating heavy metals in your body is by hair testing. There are many companies in the U.S. who will test samples of your hair for this purpose. You do not have to be present. Your doctor may use one service, your friends another. You may choose one. Otherwise you can write to such organizations which will send an application for you to sign signifying your permission, and give you exact instructions on how to send the hair sample (very important). Fees vary. I like one in particular, since it is nonprofit, reliable and reasonably quick. It is Health Evaluations whose address is found on page 45.

NOTES

1. Linda Clark, *Know Your Nutrition*. New Canaan, CT: Keats Publishing, Inc., 1973.

2. Weston A. Price, D.D.S., *Nutrition and Physical Degeneration*. La Mesa, CA: Price-Pottenger Nutrition Foundation, 1945, 1970.

3. *The Esoterian*. Vol. VI., No. 1, 1979.

4. G. A. Goldsmith, *Food and Civilization*. Springfield, IL: Charles C. Thomas, 1966, pp. 157-159.

5. M. E. Lotz, et al., 1968 *New England Journal of Medicine* 278, pp. 409-415.

6. John M. Ellis, M.D. and James Presley, *Vitamin B$_6$—The Doctor's Report*. New York: Harper and Row, 1973.

7. Broda O. Barnes, M.D. and Lawrence Galton, *Hypothyroisism: The Unsuspected Illness*. New York: Thomas Y. Crowell, 1976.

8. Carl C. Pfeiffer, Ph.D., M.D., *Zinc and Other Micronutrients*. New Canaan, CT: Keats Publishing, Inc. 1978. Paperback edition.

CHAPTER SIX

Choose Your Foods Carefully

By this time you have learned the rudiments of how good nutrition has helped to develop and maintain good health in countless people in all parts of the world. Actually, these foods are simple: whole, natural foods, containing *all* nutrients such as vitamins, minerals and protein factors (amino acids) as provided by nature, and taken from the sea where the sea water contains such a rich growing mineral medium, or from naturally highly mineralized soils. In all cases, health among the primitives was found to deteriorate when processed or fractionated foods were substituted, or synthesized, or contaminated by artificial colors and flavors resulting in poor fuel for the body machinery.

DIGESTION AND ENZYMES

It will come as no surprise then that as good as natural food can be, it still cannot provide the necessary help if you cannot digest or assimilate it. The best diet in the world is useless unless these requirements are satisfied. What can you do to insure good digestion and assimilation? One answer is to eat without tension, in order to prevent temporary paralysis of your digestive apparatus.

Recently a woman with numerous allergies told me that she was sure they were due to the fact that as she starts to eat she begins to think about all of her business problems, and as a result she tenses up and does not digest her food. This occurs in spite of the fact that her diet is well-nigh perfect as measured in the terms we have been discussing.

This means that when you sit down to eat, you should relax and think about pleasant things only. Do not allow any bickering, or negative topics (or thoughts) to take over. This applies to the entire family: father, mother, children, or you, yourself, if or when you eat alone.

ENZYMES FOR BETTER DIGESTION

The second aid to digestion is enzymes. Where do you find them? Easy: in raw foods. Your body, if it is in good condition, can also manufacture them. There are enzymes in every living being, and they occur by the thousands in all parts of your body. They serve as body catalysts, stimulators, housecleaners and facilitate the function of every cell, every gland, every organ. Enzymes also occur in foods *unless they are cooked*. This is because high heat kills enzymes, turning live food into dead food. As an example, look at the green tomato you may put on your window still to ripen. (The enzymes turn it red.) Yet if you interrupt the ripening process, by cooking it, the enzyme activity stops immediately. This applies to underripe fruit, too.

So, basically, we can get these enzymes, which add to, or replace our own enzymes, by eating raw food. Freezing does not kill enzymes; it merely inactivates them until thawing takes place. As Dr. Edward Howell, a health physician who has devoted a lifetime to the study of enzymes, says, "You may have all the nutrients—vitamins, proteins and minerals . . . but you still need the life element—the enzymes, to keep your body alive and well."[1]

But, as Dr. Howell adds, our own enzyme system may have been allowed to run down (for which there is still help available). He explains that we are endowed at birth with a large supply of enzymes, but, like money from the bank, these enzymes are rapidly depleted in the process of trying to run the body machinery: the brain, heart, kidneys, glands, lungs and other organs, and our enzyme balance account can run low. This depletion has no doubt been accentuated by eating too many cooked foods, so that our body had been required to keep the system replenished without help from sufficient enzymes in raw food, which can otherwise lighten the load.

In this case we can take added enzymes in supplement form from health food stores, to help balance the enzyme budget. If your digestion is waning, there are digestive enzymes for protein (such as *protease* and others; *lipase,* for fat digestion; *amylase* for starches; and *cellulase* for fiber or cellulose digestion). Other names may appear, but fortunately they are natural since, except for RNA, chemists today have not been able to synthesize enzymes. As one example of a natural protein digestant, papain, from papaya, is often used for human digestion problems as well as for a meat tenderizer.

IS THERE A CONNECTION BETWEEN COOKED FOODS AND POOR HEALTH?

The best answer we can find to this question is the classic study of nine hundred cats by the late Francis M. Pottenger, Jr., M.D., who fed cats both raw and cooked diets and watched the results from one generation to another. Those cats on cooked foods eventually developed every ailment common to mankind today: heart disease, kidney and thyroid ailments plus gum and teeth disturbances; also allergies, infections, diarrhea, pneumonia, loss of sex interest and fertility, and many others.[2]

In each succeeding generation, the diseases became more apparent. On the other hand, those cats on raw foods, regardless of generation, remained flexible, active, bright eyed and active. (As Dr. Howell observed, enzymes are also a contraindication to aging.) There are motion pictures of these cats in a color film available from Price Pottenger Nutrition Foundation. If you have an opportunity to see this film, don't miss it!

Enzymes are a fascinating subject. For instance, one surprise is that each enzyme occurs in the food in which it is formed by nature to help the digestion of that food. *This explains why whole foods are more important than fractionated ones.* Enzymes necessary for the digestion and assimilation of each food are in *that* whole food unless thoughtlessly or deliberately removed. A beet enzyme helps the digestion of beets; a radish or carrot enzyme helps the assimilation of that vegetable (Howell). So a raw salad will help its own digestion, not necessarily other foods eaten at the same time.

SHOULD YOU EAT A 100% RAW DIET TODAY?

Discoveries thus far indicate that some food is better for you cooked. Raw food requires a great deal of chewing to prepare it for digestion, and some people do not have adequate teeth for this purpose. In this case either light cooking, or fresh-squeezed raw juices (the latter contains all enzymes) are acceptable substitutes.

Some foods are actually better absorbed when cooked. This (with the exception of fresh juice) is true of carrots, which, when cooked have been found to release more vitamin A than raw carrots. Dr. Howell also stated in this connection, "It is not wise for the average individual to live solely on a raw diet, today." He makes this statement because of the physical, mental and emotional stress in our times and explains that wild animals living on raw foods spend much time hunting and eating such food, and the balance in rest or sleep.

Dr. Howell continues, "It is perhaps true that the pace of civilized life requires a certain amount of readily available nourishment. Because some foods are enclosed in tough, fibrous cell walls, requiring considerable time for complete digestion . . . cooked foods supply readily usable nourishment because of the fact that the heat of the cooking annihilates the cell walls."

This is where enzyme supplements come to the rescue. If you know or suspect that you have an inadequate digestive enzyme problem, by all means correct it by taking the necessary enzyme. They are clearly labelled on containers in health stores, and in some cases there are enzymes for all purposes (fat, protein, starch and cellulose) grouped in the same product. A doctor who became nutritionally converted told me, "I would not be as healthy or energetic as I am if I did not take enzymes." His energy is phenomenal.

There are many other surprises in enzymes. Vegetables and fruits contain fewer enzymes partly because an enzyme is found in a *protein* fraction[3] and partly because fruits and vegetables are more highly diluted with water (Howell).

Digestion also calls for thorough chewing of starches, since these starches need saliva (which occurs in the mouth), for proper digestion. This is not necessarily so for protein. Tests with dogs show that a piece of meat is almost instantly dissolved by hydrochloric acid in the stomach when swallowed even in large bites. However, if a person is deficient in HCl, as many are, it is extremely important that one take either the protein-digesting enzyme or HCl with pepsin, or perhaps both products as some people do.

You can conserve on your own body enzyme manufacture by taking enzymes, says Dr. Howell, who encourages you to do so. In addition to enzyme supplements, he reports that the food highest in enzymes is *sprouts*. But *don't cook them* (or yogurt-type foods either) or you lose the natural enzyme activity!

Enzymes may explain why some people, according to Dr. Kelley's metabolism tests, (mentioned in Chapter Three) have a cooked food rather than a raw food metabolism. As just explained, enzyme supplements are therefore needed if you are a "cooked food" eater instead of a "raw food" eater.

However, the need for raw food elements is not mere guesswork. The late Paul Kouchakoff, M.D., of the Institute of Clinical Chemistry, Lausanne, Switzerland, found after completing three hundred experiments that the type of food eaten immediately affects the body. He discovered that when cooked or processed food is eaten, the body's white corpuscles (which fight infection) mobilize instantly. But when raw foods, or foods in their natural state which have not been altered by heat or processing are eaten, the white corpuscles do not increase.[4] His solution, then, as confirmed by his experiments, showed that if you eat a cooked food, then add a raw food, the white corpuscles do *not* mobilize. Or, if you eat a processed food, *two* raw foods are needed to neutralize the effect of a processed food.[4]

Bircher-Benner[5] came up with the idea that if you eat your raw food, as a salad, at the beginning of a meal, it will trick the white corpuscles from activating. Some nutritionists do not buy this concept, since they believe that perhaps the warning signal may be a body protective device and should not be ignored. The Kouchakoff remedy of using one raw food for every cooked one, or two raw foods for every processed food may be safer.

FERMENTED FOODS

Fermentation is a form of preserving foods at a low cost. Such foods which also contain enzymes, are considered easy to digest due to a predigestion activity, and have been proved also to contain certain other health benefits, including an ability to improve the intestinal flora; an aid in constipation; and in the case of yogurt, to provide a natural antibiotic against infections.

The Orient is centuries ahead of us in making and using fermented foods which are common in China, Japan, the Philippines and other Asian countries. They ferment vegetables; the Chinese and Japanese ferment bean curd (tofu) and soy sauce from soy beans, and the Japanese make a marvelous miso, a fermented soybean paste which is added to chicken or other broth used with rice and served as a soup in Japan for breakfast. You have to eat this delicacy to appreciate it.

America's favorite fermented foods include sauerkraut, kosher dill pickles, made with salt and spices, dill, garlic, and *no vinegar* (if truly authentic), sourdough bread, rolls and others such as the famous sheepherders flapjacks. Even though the sourdough products are cooked, the enzymes have done their work in predigestion of ingredients and they are still considered good for you.

Beatrice Trum Hunter in her two little paperback books[6,7] has given complete directions for making fermented foods, including sauerkraut. There are two methods of fermenting: using layers of rock salt (ice cream salt usually) interlayered with vegetables; or covering the vegetables with a salty brine. In either case the ratio of salt to water must be exact, and the foods should be kept completely submerged during the fermenting period (which ranges from weeks to months) for successful results. If you are interested in learning the secrets of this inexpensive successful type of food preparation, these two booklets will give you all the help you need. I must also recommend recipes for traditional kosher dill pickles and for marvelous mustard contained in the *Guide to Living Foods*.[8] Following is a general recipe for sauerkraut.[9]

SAUERKRAUT RECIPE

This recipe is simple:

Cut cabbage fine with a sharp knife.

Using a nonmetal crock, build up alternating layers of cabbage and rock or kosher salt (available at most groceries and supermarkets). Push the whole mixture down and cover with a plate, topped with a weight in order to keep the sauerkraut submerged in the juices which will soon develop.

Cover the crock with a clean cloth to keep out insects and dust. Store in a cool, dark place. Fermentation will take longer in winter than in summer. You can establish when it is "ready" by the taste and the consistency you like.

For a recipe without salt, or for "raw" sauerkraut made in ordinary glass canning jars, see *Guide to Living Foods*.[8]

Mrs. Hunter's book on yogurt and other fermented beverages is excellent, with full documentation for all claims made. Unfortunately, the newest, easiest addition to her parade of fermented milks became available after the publication of her book. This particular milk ferment is easier to make than yogurt since it does not require heating, but does ferment at room temperature, to be followed by placing it in the refrigerator to increase firmness. It is a very mild, subtle and delicious drink and the starter is a Finnish import, called Piima, pronounced *Peema:* it is available in this country only from Piima, P.O. Box 2116, La Mesa, CA 92041

Piima is made of an herb, called Butterwort, and was discovered when it was learned that the milk of cows who grazed on it clabbered at room temperature. Piima is delicious as a drink, or it can be made into a natural custard, party Bavarian, ice cream or a milk shake. The Scandinavian women even rub it on their faces to help remove wrinkles. Like yogurt it is perpetuated by using a starter from the previous batch to begin a new one. It is both delicate and delicious.

FOOD INTOLERANCES

Should everyone, on reading this book take their first step toward better eating by using whole wheat or other whole grain bread and cereals? The answer is *absolutely not!*

As good as these foods are for the majority, for the minority they may be very bad! For some people eating the whole grains, even whole wheat, is the equivalent to eating poison. This reaction is not considered an allergy, which can be a fleeting, come-and-go-disturbance, but an *intolerance* which is far more serious. It indicates a breakdown somewhere in the body mechanism, a condition which may be genetic or due to unknown causes, but which is an aberration or malfunction of that body, just as color blindness is a condition some people are born with. Food intolerances, however, are more common than suspected; often the victim is unaware of the problem.

Recently, there have been some gushing news reports that the the use of white bread is giving way to a greater use of whole wheat bread. This is fine for those who can use wheat but many can't. Lloyd Rosenvold, M.D., has pointed out in his book on high blood pressure[10] that those with a wheat intolerance are courting disaster by eating it in any form. He gives the example of a patient whose systolic pressure shot up from normal to 230 within six hours after eating wheat! One major medical clinic, known the world over, (whose name cannot be divulged) believes that wheat is the No. 1 intolerance factor in the world. Some wheat intolerants dare not touch wheat germ, wheat germ oil, or even vitamin E (if it is derived from wheat germ oil). A dry E or that taken from vegetable oils would be safer in this case. I have seen wheat intolerants break out in an angry rash a short time after taking wheat germ. Symptoms vary. I am a wheat intolerant myself and I can assure you it is not worth taking chances with.

Others who are more seriously afflicted with wheat intolerance, even intolerant of rye, barley and oats may have a predisposition toward multiple sclerosis, or celiac disease. The cause has been found to be *gluten,* a sticky substance in these grains which holds bread together. The best description of these diseases I have found, which are similar to each other and apparently due to the same cause, is in an excellent book about the serious effects of gluten.[11]

Here again we face the problem of individual difference, which, though in this case is in the minority, is still tragic. Everyone should be aware of this problem, if not for oneself, for a friend or family member.

ANOTHER INTOLERANCE WORLDWIDE

Fortunately, although wheat and whole grains (actually gluten, one factor in these grains) affects only the minority, another food affects the majority. This intolerance is cow's milk. Of course these are fighting words to the dairy industry, but they are true, nevertheless. Many people have already discovered their own milk intolerance; others have not. The cause is an inborn aberration, the absence of an important enzyme, *lactase,* which is needed to assimilate *lactose* or milk sugar. Babies who have been breast-fed usually start life with an adequate supply of lactase. But on weaning it disappears, apparently for the remainder of life for those people who are countless. The symptoms of intolerance of cow's milk and its products are usually intestinal gas, cramps and abnormal mucus.

Some people can bypass this intolerance by using goat's milk, or soy milk. For others, soy milk, in particular, is disturbing, since it, too, causes flatulence (gas) as well as edema (water storage) in some people.

Happily, after years of search, a solution to cow's milk intolerance has recently been found. A tablet has been formulated to replace the missing lactase, and those who take it *before* using milk, cheese or other dairy products disturbing to them, are helped. This product is available in health stores and is called milk digestant.

This milk intolerance protective *tablet* is my favorite since it really does the job if taken according to direction. Since I am also a cow's milk intolerant, but can use goat's milk, I know whereof I speak; this product has been a lifesaver to me as well as to numerous others who have written me. Some competitive products treat the milk, not the person. The tablets are, in my opinion far more convenient than adding the lactase enzymes to the milk which requires twenty-four hours for refrigeration to complete the lactase culture. Also when I eat out, I can take my tablets with me.[12]

NOTES

1. Linda Clark, "Enzymes Can Help Your Health," *Let's LIVE* Magazine, June, 1977.

2. Linda Clark, *Stay Young Longer.* New York: Pyramid Publications, 1968. Paperback edition.
also,
American Journal of Orthodontics and Oral Surgery, August, 1946.

3. Harrow-Mazur, *Textbook of Biochemistry.* Philadelphia: W. B. Saunders, 1958.

4. Paul Kouchakoff, M.D., "The Influence of Cooked Food on the Blood Formula of Man," (excerpted from Proceedings of the First International Congress of Microbiology, Paris, 1930). *Guide to Living Foods,* La Mesa, CA: Price-Pottenger Nutrition Foundation, pp. 7-8.

5. Ralph Bircher, "A Turning Point in Nutritional Science" reprint No. 80, Milwaukee, WI: Lee Foundation for Nutritional Research.

6. Beatrice Trum Hunter, *Fact-Book on Fermented Foods and Beverages.* New Canaan, CT: Keats Publishing, Inc., 1973.

7. Beatrice Trum Hunter, *Fact-Book on Yogurt, Kefir and Other Milk Cultures.* New Canaan, CT: Keats Publishing, Inc., 1973.

8. *Guide to Living Foods.* Price-Pottenger Nutrition Foundation.

9. Linda Clark, "Creative Barter," *Let's LIVE* Magazine, May, 1977, p.12.

10. Lloyd Rosenvold, M.D., *Drop Your Blood Pressure,* New York: Harcourt Brace/Jove.

11. Hilda Cherry Hills, *Good Food: Gluten-Free,* New Canaan, CT: Keats Publishing, Inc., 1976.

12. Linda Clark, "Outwitting Food Intolerances," *Let's LIVE* Magazine, August, 1977.

CHAPTER SEVEN

How and When to Take Supplements and Tips on Salt

Good food is better than supplements taken alone. As a nutrition reporter, Rebecca Kirby, wisely stated, "The food one eats (or should eat) is the primary source of the life supporting nutrients."[1]

The real reason for taking supplements is to compensate for those nutrients which have been removed from food or soil or to compensate for any deficiency you may have acquired due to an inadequate diet. Nutritional doctors may begin by giving you supplements in mega (large) potencies until you have overcome your deficiencies. Then supplements usually should be gradually diminished while food quality is increased. If a high supplement potency is continued too long, for many it may prove detrimental and over stimulating to the body, similar to whipping a tired horse.

Here are some general rules for taking supplements.

1. Don't worry about them. You may be doing more harm than good by tensing up as you wonder if you are taking the right vitamin at the wrong time.

2. In general, supplements (if not completely synthetic) come from food, so should be taken with or immediately after food. This applies to vitamins, minerals and digestants.

3. Because supplements are usually concentrated, they should not be taken on an empty stomach.

4. Some stimulating vitamins, such as vitamin A, and for some people, vitamin E, should be taken mornings rather than evenings when they might interfere with sleep.

From time to time announcements of antagonism between certain vitamins and other nutrients are announced. Watch for them and give them serious consideration. For example, Wilfrid E. Shute, M.D., the vitamin E specialist, tells us that *inorganic* iron and female hormones taken simultaneously with vitamin E interfere with the vitamin E assimilation. To bypass this problem, he advises taking one item in the morning and the other at night, separating the two antagonists by eight to twelve hours. For example, you could take vitamin E for breakfast and *inorganic* iron (synthetic, chemical iron) or the female hormones at dinner. *Natural iron from food is not a problem* since it often appears together with vitamin E naturally in growing foods.

SHOULD YOU AVOID COMBINING CERTAIN FOODS?

I questioned several nutritionists about avoiding certain other food combinations and the general consensus was that this was possibly an individual, not a common problem. In fact, often some of these very same food combinations grow or appear together in nature. It is possible that there may be an enzyme deficiency (as explained in the previous chapter). If you are suffering from a digestive disturbance, it may be due to one food only, instead of a combination. Or you may wish to experiment with various enzyme digestants in order to solve your problem. There is no danger involved—and you may find a solution. Perhaps you lack a protein digesting enzyme or a fat digester, both of which problems might be eliminated by taking the correct digestant. However, for some people, avoiding certain combinations of foods is the answer. This is discussed in detail in Chapter Fourteen.

A SALT-FREE DIET?

Nothing raises my hackles more than the indiscriminate parroting of the admonition to cut down on salt or avoid it altogether.

I hear on all sides the statement which appears in newspapers and magazines, that too much salt is dangerous. *It depends on the salt!* Recent research shows that in general it is not so much a problem of cutting down or out salt but of eliminating the *type* of salt which causes danger!

Salt apparently is a family or complex somewhat similar to the B complex, or the C complex, known as the bioflavonoids. The sodium family is similar. Table salt usually contains one factor only—except for an antimoisturizer. This factor is *sodium chloride,* only one factor of the salt family, and the real mischief maker. This factor, it is true, has been found implicated with water storage (edema), high blood pressure and other disturbances. On the other hand, *whole salt* or the entire salt family includes other factors too: all the trace minerals most people need. Whole salt originally comes from the sea, or in some cases from land salt mines. But this whole salt is good for you—in moderation—not as dangerous as sodium chloride alone which is sold in regular groceries and is on the tables of most homes.

Getting whole salt has become a real problem. No one seems to know why.

Several years ago a company which was producing whole natural sea salt in this country was closed down by government authorities. About that time a biochemistry student, doing his Ph.D. thesis at a major university, wrote me that he had analyzed salt from supermarkets as well as from many health stores. Both were labelled "sea salt," but all of it was, he said, pure sodium chloride only.

Why? When salt from sea water is dried, the sodium chloride in large amounts is precipitated and separated from the delicate, minute trace minerals which are often thrown away. The sodium chloride is then boxed and sold as table salt. Another case of a fractionated food! It did indeed, come from the sea originally, but, OH, what has happened to it since then!

Natural ocean water has long been used by physicians as a substitute for blood transfusions when blood was unavailable. This is because the chemical analysis of sea water and blood is nearly identical. So it must be safe![2]

Josef Isser, M.D., a German physician, writes, "Commercial salt . . . is almost pure sodium chloride. It is not balanced with calcium, potassium, and magnesium, and other trace elements, and is undesirable from a health point of view. [Water from inland seas is usually too highly concentrated and often contaminated.]

"In preference, . . . safe, whole ocean sea salt should be used because it contains all the necessary salt substances *in a mixture similar to that found in blood.*

"But even sea salts from the sea should not be used to excess. If there is an exaggerated desire for salt, it should be counteracted by using forms of green herbs and seasonings of high biological value."[2] (Such seasonings are available in health food stores.

A list of acceptable whole salts and their sources follows.

(This list may change but at this writing the following natural salts are available.)

For those who want the imported whole sea salt ask health stores to order Natural Sea Salt from France: Erewhon Products, Cambridge ME 02141.

Health stores can also order:

Indian Mound Natural Table Salt—a land salt from Bald Mountain Formulations, P. O. Box 147, Mineral Wells, TX 76067

• De Sousa's *Salt of the Earth,* a land mined organic rock salt can be ordered from De Sousa's Organic Farm, Box 1114, San Jacinto, CA 92383. This can be pulverized in a blender or small grinder for table use.

Health stores usually already carry herb salt seasonings or herb salt substitutes. One which combines *sea salt and herbs* is called Herba-Mare, from Switzerland. Stores may order from *Bioforce of America, Ltd.,* Westbury, NY 11590.

Kosher rock salt is acceptable and available at supermarkets but must be home ground for table use.

Meanwhile I am told there is a government edict that all salt sold in this country *must* contain at least 90% or more sodium chloride! What is going on?

Also, I am told that it is now legal to sell only whole salt unless it is rock salt, which would mean you would probably have to pulverize it in a blender, too inconvenient for most people, and therefore more unlikely to sell as well as preground sodium chloride.

Some sea salt has been exposed to extremely high temperatures which destroy the delicate trace minerals, again leaving only the single sodium chloride residue. Whole salt tastes and looks exactly like table salt (sodium chloride). Any biochemistry textbook will tell you that the body's electrical system needs salt to generate body electricity! In fact I have talked with a few doctors who know this and urge whole salt for their patients. One doctor told me that a patient had been sent to the hospital by another doctor for a brain scan, expecting a possible heart attack and stroke, only to find the patient low in sodium! Many people who are dragging from fatigue, this doctor told me often do so merely because of sodium deficiency. We all know, of course, the "heat stroke" effects of salt loss through perspiration during hot weather, a condition for which salt is used as a remedy.

But this is not the only need for salt. Adelle Davis[3] states that a deficiency in sodium due to exhausted adrenals can cause muscle weakness. The remedy, she said, is to eat more salty foods. Salt is also needed by the body to help manufacture HCl—the protein digestant.

Salt is one of the acquired tastes—it can be habit forming, so don't overdo it. But when you do eat salt, now that you know the difference, choose the right kind—whole salt, and use it in moderation. There are whole salts such as kosher salt available at supermarkets, and a greater selection in health stores if you know what to look for.

NOTES

1. Linda Clark, *Know Your Nutrition*. New Canaan, CT: Keats Publishing, Inc., 1973, p. 6.

2. Josef Isser, M.D., *Cancer, A Second Opinion*. London: Hodder and Stoughton, 1975.

3. Adelle Davis, *Let's Get Well*. New York: New American Library, Inc., 1972.

CHAPTER EIGHT

Important Diet Information on Sugar, Honey, Fats and Beverages

WHAT IS WRONG WITH SUGAR?

Is the case against sugar exaggerated?

I believe that for a seasoning, a pinch of sugar here or there is not going to do you in. But when sugar is used in large amounts as a *food,* it displaces other better, more nutritious foods and can cause real trouble. Jim Wallace, an assistant professor of the University of Mexico, and a worker in the field of rehabilitation therapy for the physically and mentally handicapped, has co-authored, with his wife, Maureen, a well-documented booklet on the effects of refined white sugar. The joint research of this couple has turned up some devastating information you should know to protect your own health as well as that of your family, particularly of your children who in this era are fast becoming *sugarholics.*[1]

The Wallaces provide this definition of refined white sugar: "Processing involves treating the sugar cane or sugar beets with a variety of toxic chemicals and gases to produce white crystals. The processing procedure also strips the raw material of any and all valuable vitamins, minerals and proteins it might have had, to provide a refined sweetener *with absolutely no nutrients.* (italics mine)[1]

Natural sugar cane on the other hand contains all the vitamins and minerals provided by nature. Man, by commercially refining the sugar cane, has produced another fractionated food! Proof: children living in countries where sugar cane grows chew on the natural, raw sugar cane and have no cavities. Children and adults elsewhere who eat the refined sugar not only have been victims of tooth decay but of the following ailments:[1]

- myopia (nearsightedness)
- learning disabilities in children
- fatigue
- hyperactivity (particularly in children)
- behavior problems, mental disturbance, schizophrenia
- violence
- alcoholism (studies show that animals fed excessive refined sugar prefer alcohol, as compared with those on a balanced diet)
- auto accident proneness
- cardiovascular disease
- arthritis

Hypoglycemia, which is the opposite of diabetes, but is often a forerunner of diabetes, are both often caused by too much sugar, which abuses the pancreas.

Refined sugar also leaches B vitamins from the body. (B vitamins help control the nervous system.)[2] Beware of that sweet tooth! I know a man who, after every meal says with a sanctimonious expression on his face, "I *always* end every meal with something sweet." A study showed that some people who ate an otherwise good diet but regularly added a sugary dessert, often developed a nervous breakdown.[2] I later learned that his sanctimonious expression was due to the fact that he had switched from alcohol (he had been an alcoholic) to sugar; he told everyone who would listen that he was a reformed alcoholic. He did not realize he now was a sugarholic, and like others, it contributed to his later breakdown.

Sugar is exactly that: a habit. The more you have, the more you want. But the reverse can also be true. You can wean yourself from a sugar craving simply by cutting it down gradually until you no longer crave it. Fresh raw fruits can be substituted for cakes, pies and cookies, but even that carries a hazard, as you will see.

WHAT ABOUT FRUCTOSE?

A young friend of mine was a fruit addict. He rented some property which had been planted with every known fruit tree species by a nationally known fruit nursery. When the trees began producing fruit my friend went absolutely berserk. He ate fruit morning, noon, and night until suddenly he began to feel unwell, and wondered why. He met another young man from Indonesia who had traveled the same overindulgent fruit route and had also become ill. Together they figured out the cause: too much fruit sugar, which the pancreas was unable to handle.

Many believe that fructose, a fruit sugar now available in supplemental form, should be better for them than glucose, or ordinary sugar. Fructose has been found to be many times sweeter than glucose and has led to serious trouble for some people, especially in hypoglycemics, partly because it can perpetuate a "sweet tooth" and create a craving for more sugar.

I am sure you understand hypoglycemia, which is also known as low blood sugar, but which is misunderstood by many, even doctors. These doctors who prescribe a candy bar to people who become fatigued easily do not realize that when sugar is consumed it does indeed raise the blood sugar and energy level temporarily. But almost immediately afterward, because it has given the pancreas a false stimulus, the blood sugar plummets downward and the person either feels irritable and lower in energy than before, or gets the "shakes" or may even black out. Eating some protein is far more successful when you feel a craving for sugar. The energy effect of protein last longer. Next time try nuts or sunflower seeds instead of sugar.

Dr. Price's natives ate very few sweets, even few natural fruits; raw fruits should probably be limited to two only, per day.

WHAT SUGAR SUBSTITUTES ARE SAFE?

Of course you know by this time that the sugar substitutes known as the cyclamates, and others, even saccharin, have been found dangerous. Are there *any* safe sugar substitutes?

There is a natural sweetener, a rice syrup, made of rice and barley now available at health stores. This could serve in small amounts as a temporary substitute for sugar. You could also use fruit in moderation, but the real solution to the problem is to wean yourself from the sweet craving as soon as possible.

There is no shortcut out of this dilemma except to learn to live with less sugar by weaning yourself gradually so that you no longer have a sugar craving (and it can be done). You will reach the point where favorite sweets you originally cherished can become sickeningly sweet to you. Kay Munson, an Iowa State University Extension nutritionist, says, "No form of sugar is better for you than any other.

"To your body, honey is hardly different than refined white sugar although it does contain trace amounts of iron and B vitamins but certainly not enough to provide a significant amount of these nutrients."[9]

However, there is another side to the honey story.

ABOUT HONEY

Much criticism of honey has recently appeared in the press. Perhaps the sugar industry is concerned about a large segment of the public shifting from white sugar to honey, which may explain some of the derogatory remarks made about honey, but not all. There is some justification about concern over honey, as you will see.

I am going to give you both sides of the story and let you decide if honey is for you. Don't jump to conclusions before reading the whole story. In this research I learned much about honey I had not known previously. My guess is that you will, too.

As previously stated, there are a few more nutrients in honey than in white sugar (which has none), but apparently these nutrients do not explain many of the good effects of honey on health. Like sea water, the scientists have not yet been able to identify all the unknown ingredients in honey.

As you know, honey has been extolled in the Bible, but newer information has been learned since Biblical times. Here are some of the reports:

- No bacteria can live in honey.[4,5] The Russians have confirmed this. The following examples were supplied by the U.S. Bureau of Entomology, which compared the results of honey with penicillin and other antibiotics.[5]

On honey:
- the dysentery germ died within 48 hours
- chronic broncho-pneumonia germs were vanquished in four days
- the peritonitis germ (which may also cause typhoid) disappeared on the fifth day

One person, a victim of "Montezuma's Revenge," (a tourist acquired diarrhea in foreign countries, particularly Mexico) reported a reversal of the disturbance by using sage honey as a remedy.

OTHER BENEFITS OF HONEY

- a stimulant to muscles and heart[6]
- an aid for anemia.[6]
- since honey is predigested by bees, it has served in some cases as a human digestive aid,preventing intestinal fermentation, discouraging flatulence (gas) and increasing intestinal activity.[6]
- has strengthened bladder function in some children who were bed wetters as well as in some elderly.[6]
- may improve memory.[6]
- an aid for catarrh and asthma, as well as a tendency toward chronic colds and hay fever.[6]
- raw honey plus propolis (the "bee glue" of the honey comb) have been found effective for various allergies.[6]
- congested sinuses have been helped by chewing bee cappings which apparently shrink mucous membranes.[6]
- used for sore throats and coughs particularly when combined with lemon juice.

- used for polio[6]
- intestinal ulcers.[6]
- nerves[6]
- insomnia.[6]
- rheumatism and arthritis.[6,7] [Honey contains the Wulzen factor (an anti-stiffness substance)][7]
- honey is also said to aid the thyroid and make calcium better available to the bones.[7]

Barbara Cartland, the English writer, tells of a woman who had been a long-time wheelchair invalid and suffered excruciating pain from arthritis. After adding honey to each meal she became pain-free, was able to discard her wheelchair and walk normally.[6]

- History has long cited the good effects of honey on male virility as confirmed by countless couples.[6,7]

HONEY FOR EXTERNAL HEALING

- Infections on skin. One infected, painful finger escaped lancing when honey was applied on a bandage. The poison was withdrawn by the honey and healing was evident in 24 hours.[6] Roman soldiers, aware of the germicidal effects of honey, used it on wounds, bruises and other injuries.[7]
- burns have become pain-free and healed rapidly with honey applications[8,6]
- boils and other infections have responded to honey applied topically.[6]

Honey has long been used as a cosmetic for firming skin and removing wrinkles.

It has also been credited with rejuvenation. C. E. Burtis tells in his book of a seventy-six-year old man in India who took a course in rejuvenation. He was bowed, aging and emaciated. He entered a darkened room on the banks of the Ganges where honey was included as part of his diet. He remained there for twelve days after which he emerged upright, looking about twenty years younger. His spider-web wrinkles were gone. No one recognized him.[7]

In addition to meditation and rest, his diet consisted of milk, honey, butter and Aonia. Others have repeated his successful experiment. In this case, it is true that honey was not used alone but was an important part of the diet. Meditation, even visualization, may well have played an important part in this transformation, too. (I do not know what Aonia is, but am searching for it. If you know, please advise me by letter in care of the publisher)

Now, after hearing of all the many benefits of honey, before you decide to take it, listen further: Here is some information on the other side of the coin.

Dr. T. L. Cleave, in his book[4] states that honey may be as dangerous as sugar *for some people.* He points out that even in the Bible, Solomon warned against eating too much honey. (Proverbs XXV 27)

Even though the sweetness factor in honey is levulose, which is assimilated slowly by the body, the fact is that it *may* upset the pancreas and "fool" it into overproduction of insulin. Though said not to be a deterrent in diabetes, many doctors do not take chances. If they allow a diabetic patient to use any sweet at all, they usually prescribe Tupelo honey, considered safer for diabetics.

Raw honey, particularly comb honey, seems to be used with special success. Barbara Cartland gave it night and morning to her husband to heal his serious bronchitis. He had lost one lung as a result of an injury in World War I, and suffered for years in hospitals from bronchitis in the remaining lung until Barbara took him home and fed him the raw honeycomb twice daily.

Each person should find his or her own way with honey, by learning the amount which does not raise the blood sugar, or make one feel worse rather than better. While it is true that honey has been found to contain the minerals: calcium, phosphorus, iron, copper, magnesium, sodium, silica and potassium as well as the B complex vitamins, there are still unknown ingredients which have not been identified. Even a few doctors have admitted that though they do not know what in honey accomplishes the good effects for some people, they say, "whatever it contains—it works!"

It is wise to use honey in the most natural possible form. Susan

Smith Jones[5] warns that one should read labels. She adds that the label should not merely say "uncooked" but should say "unheated." "Uncooked" is a term legally allowed for processing at 160° F to destroy some ingredients. Crystallization is not to be shunned. It does not mean spoilage, but rather may be proof of lack of applied heat. Beatrice Trum Hunter advises one to buy the honey which has the words, "raw" and "unfiltered" on the label.[3] Don't trust the term, "organic." It may or may not be true.

Heating for clarification so that honey becomes bright and clear enough to read the label through it, means that nutrients have been removed. University of Minnesota studies also found that clarifying honey removed vitamins.[3] Cloudy honey is more inclined to be natural. So don't fall for the terms "pure," or "deluxe." The greater the tampering the less nutritious.

Probably the greatest disadvantage of honey is that it perpetuates the desire for sweets, and though comb honey is usually recommended only in a one teaspoon dosage (at a time), it still may start you on a habit of again wanting sweets, once you have weaned yourself from sugar, which may spill over to using more sugar and other sweeteners. It may or may not upset the blood sugar level of many people. So, I repeat, it is not an innocent addition to your diet if it disagrees with you. Use it sparingly at first. If it does disagree with you, blame yourself, not the honey.

If it helps you, by all means make use of it, as many doctors will agree.

If you do find that you can use honey safely and have the will power to limit its use, as Solomon suggested, you can substitute a minimum of honey for sugar in baked goods or cooking on a one to one basis (one cup or less of honey instead of one cup of sugar, but decrease the amount of liquids accordingly in the recipe since honey contains water). Because of this, baked goods made with honey remain moist longer than those made with sugar.

But the possible danger of the effect of honey on the pancreas (in some people) and the possibility of activating your sweet tooth are not the only hazards. The following shocker tells the rest of the story of honey. In this case you can blame the honey.

Colonel Clair, President of Hawaii Bee Keepers Association, in a radio station interview, stated that all honey contains pesticide residues, "there'd be no way to avoid that from nectar collected from plants which have been sprayed with pesticides . . . California loses up to one-fourth of its beehives each year due to pesticide applications. [The Beekeepers Idemnity Payment Program pays beekeepers for bees killed by pesticides used near their apiaries, but the beekeeper must prove the kill was due to pesticides.] The money for pesticide spraying comes from our tax dollar, despite the fact that it was the chemical companies who committed the deed.

"Not only do bees bring in $23,500,000 per year in bee hive products, they also bring in, indirectly, the $600-million agricultural crops that are pollinated by them . . . I deal with nature—and beekeeping as it applies to nature. Bees are essential to our present way of life. Our dairy industry, poultry industry and most of our fruits and vegetables, nuts and legumes depend on pollination. I don't think the general public has been aware of this . . . The problem hasn't been appreciated until recently, and the scope of it, still isn't appreciated. What opened up many farmers' eyes—and minds— was that regardless of how much insecticides/pesticides they used, the insects developed resistance, and the chemical companies developed stronger pesticides. The insects again develop resistance, and all of the predator insects are killed off. The cotton crops were almost wiped out, until farmers . . . found that natural biological controls were far more effective. The entire pesticide program has been a failure. Not that you can't produce a fruit, vegetable, or grain, with the use of pesticides, but is it safe to eat?

"In general, chemical agriculture is failing, and there's concern, not only in this country, but USSR, India, Africa, where they're having severe problems . . . The foods we eat no longer contain adequate nourishment—a person couldn't chew up enough in a day to nourish himself.

"When a carrot that's supposed to have from 10,000 to 100,000 units of Vitamin A, and has 500 to 1,000—there's something wrong in the carrot patch. Much of the food sold today has nothing to do with nutritive quality—it is sold purely on appearance. Fruits and vegetables are raised and picked get to market only on the basis of cosmetic appearance. If they were sold according to nutritional content, most of them would have to be garbaged. If they were labelled according to pesticide concentration, they'd rot on the shelf. It's becoming obvious to anyone who wants to look into the facts—that the only way out is going to be "organic" agriculture—returning all of the vegetable matter to the soil. There's a world of difference in the mineral and vitamin content in vegetables and fruits when they're grown naturally. Naturally composed gardens could probably get the vitamin and mineral content they need, providing the garden is not in a polluted atmosphere.

". . . In Hawaii all of the bees are placed upwind of any commercial farming activity . . . Honey from an area that isn't exposed to residues, to the extent that California is, would be cleaner . . . We don't feed sugar to our bees nor do we feed them any drugs . . . The California beekeeper feeds sugar syrup, white cane sugar syrup or reclaimed candy (this unsold candy is melted down and made into a syrup feed, full of colorings and other chemicals) then before the spring blossoms start, he begins feeding either dried pollen or some mixture of protein substances to stimulate brood-rearing . . . They're all artificially supported by dry milk powder and soybean concoctions and/or dried pollen and sugar syrup.

"For some strange reason, the bees fed this way develop all kinds of illnesses. It is a tremendous puzzle to the USDA. They have six research labs through the U.S. working on this . . . obviously, the solution is to drug them. They feed them a sulfa drug or terramycin. The residues of these drugs go into the honey, and there have been good research reports, good medical papers, showing the residual amounts of tetracycline in honey . . . some poor soul who's taking tetracycline for some other problem gets an extra dose in some honey and you can imagine the side effects. These drugs are fed usually in the spring and then in the fall, just to insure that these bees are adequately drugged." [We're doing the same thing to bees that we've done to cows, pigs, and people—drugging to treat the symptoms—ignoring the cause of the trouble.]

(Reprinted by permission)
Of the *Esoterian*
May 1979

ARE RAW SUGARS OK?

What about those so-called raw sugars available in various stores? According to Dave Ajay, president of The National Nutritional Foods Association (health stores), writing in *Health Food Retailing* (January, 1979) these raw sugars are not the equivalent of nature's unprocessed sugar. Ajay takes a dim view of them. It is said that in some cases, white sugar is merely colored brown by adding molasses. However, Ajay has discovered a totally natural, unprocessed raw sugar cane crystals from Nicaragua, which health stores may order, provided the political unrest in that country has not interfered with their exports) from Green Earth Enterprises, 2741 South Compton Avenue, Los Angeles, California.

Like alcohol, coffee and certain drugs, sugar is an addictive substance. How does this addiction start? Often through parents who wheedle their children into eating their vegetables by rewarding them with a sweet dessert.

Don't forget, too, that an addiction for sweets can begin in school. As everyone knows (except some parents) many children hoard their lunch money only to buy a candy bar, or a sweet soft drink at the nearest store. Fortunately parents are awakening to the threat of sugared cereals extolled in TV commercials, and are substituting something more wholesome. A wise mother I know promised her children that if they would bring home any sweet given them elsewhere she would trade it for something they liked very much. (Popcorn, a wholesome food, sunflower seeds or nuts are possibilities). Now those children have perpetuated the same method with *their* children.

FATS—WHICH ONES ARE ACCEPTABLE?

We all need some fat in the diet to help the assimilation of the fat soluble vitamins A, D, E, and K. These vitamins accomplish many benefits including better vision, a sheen for skin and hair, and more efficient calcium assimilation for stronger bones, teeth and nerves.

Remember, too, the model who could not lose weight until she added some vegetable oil to her daily diet, yet many people avoid fat for fear of gaining weight. Vegetable oils are beginning to be questioned because of the rough processing to which they are subjected. What formerly was considered "cold pressed" oil is no longer that. Due to heating of seeds before oil is pressed, or due to extreme pressure of machinery used for pressing the oil, not only is great heat generated but oil is also separated from its synergists.[10] Again, this represents a fractionated food, thus is less healthful or less well utilized than it should be.

Not only that, the theory of saturated fats versus unsaturated fats is losing favor. The newer idea is to use soft fats, such as butter, (which melt at body temperature) rather than fats which are artifically hardened by hydrogenation. Hydrogenation, a synthetic process of hardening fats, is still suspect and unnatural. (Lard and margarine are examples.)

Instead of wrenching the oils away from the seeds, you can eat the raw seeds, whole or in sprouted form, which supply the oil naturally and is preferable. If you must have an oil for salad dressing, there are several alternatives: sesame oil is supposed to be less processed, thus more natural; and olive oil is not a vegetable oil at all, but a fruit oil! It is made from the olive fruit, not seeds, thus acceptable.

After opening a bottle of any kind of oil, refrigerate it immediately to prevent oxidation (which produces rancidity). Since vitamin E is an anti-oxidizer, to prevent rancidity, pierce several capsules of vitamin E oil (in 100 or 200 I.U.'s) and add them to the oil before refrigerating.

Still another alternative is to grind your own oil bearing seeds in a blender or other small grinder, and add, with desired flavorings, to tomato or other juice. This can make a unique as well as delicious and healthful salad dressing!

Dr. Francis Pottenger, Jr., of the famous cat studies, recommended animal fats, rather than vegetable fats. He suggested using the animal fats found around organ meats of properly fed animals, or fish, fish roe, and poultry.

Dr. Price preferred raw cream, butter, cod-liver oil, and bone marrow instead of manufactured fats.

THE MYSTERIOUS "ACTIVATOR X"

Dr. Price, when he was conducting his tribal studies, discovered a mysterious substance he called "Factor X," which he observed present in high vitamin summer butter, seafoods and animal oils such as seal and cod-liver oil. This mysterious Factor X which still has not been completely identified, was tested in Dr. Price's laboratory on his return home. Although we do not yet know all foods which contain it, Factor X has been found to be a health promoter and contains at least ten times more fat soluble vitamin and mineral activators than ordinary foods, according to the Price laboratory tests. Scientists who are aware of Factor X are still searching for further food sources of it. It was present in nearly every primitive diet.

Meanwhile, Dr. Price discovered that the presence of Factor X improved mineral utilization, and immunity to dental caries (cavities). Wherever this factor was high, heart disease and pneumonia were lowest. As a result of 20,000 tests on dairy products in five different countries, he found "Activator X" was related to sunshine and green fodder (fresh, raw, or quickly dried) for grazing animals. The nutrient appeared to be a fat soluble substance, yet was not vitamin D. He named it Activator X or Factor X. He found it highest in dairy products such as summer butter, cream, fish and cod-liver oil. In his book, *Nutrition and Physical Degeneration,* Dr. Price tells of two cases where health was incredibly improved by the use of Activator X, as an adjunct to other whole foods.[11]

One was a case of a four-year-old boy of a poor family whose parents had called the minister to baptize him due to impending death. The child had a broken leg in a cast, and suffered from convulsions. He also had serious dental caries as well. His ailments had persisted for eight months without improvement. His diet had included skim milk and white flour. Dr. Price prescribed a diet of whole milk, a gruel of whole, freshly ground wheat, topped with a dessert spoon of high vitamin butter oil plus cod-liver oil to supply added Activator X. After the first meal, the child slept through the night for the first time in eight months without a convulsion. Six weeks later when the minister paid him a visit, the child was jumping over a fence.

Another child, five years old, was even worse off. He suffered from acute pain, arthritis, rheumatic fever, severe dental caries and heart disease. He was bedfast, and cried for hours. A similar diet was prescribed at the request of the parents, and fresh ground or cracked wheat and oats plus whole milk and cod-liver oil, as well as sources of Activator X dairy products from animals which grazed on green pastures. The boy's swollen joints disappeared, pain and crying stopped. He slept soundly and gained weight. Pictures in the book show his progress.[11]

The scientific search for additional foods containing Activator X still continues. Without realizing it, most primitives consumed this Factor X or Activator X in their diet.

BEVERAGES—WHICH ARE BEST?

Individual differences were never more in the spotlight, because of charges made against certain beverages.

Alcohol is one, yet doctors often allow a three ounce glass of wine for many elderly people *with their evening meal* as a natural tranquilizer and something to look forward to in an otherwise bleak existence. But don't kid yourself, it is as easy to keep drinking wine and become a "wino" as it is to become an alcoholic. Furthermore, a British medical journal says red wine may cause headache and depression.[12]

Since coffee contains niacin, a B vitamin which stimulates circulation, some people, including doctors, insist that a minimum of *one cup* of coffee *with breakfast,* is a must for them. If you can get by with it, cheers! If you feel shaky later, it is not for you. Forget it. Both alcohol and coffee will be discussed at greater length in Chapter XII.

WATER

For those who tell you never to drink water with your meals, I say Phooey! Some people have throat muscle tightness or congestion and cannot swallow food without a sip of water now and then. Cold water relaxes the throat muscles, if needed. So, if you are thirsty, drink water. Your body may be telling you something. Consider your own needs before those of prophets of doom.

WHAT TO EXPECT FROM YOUR NEW DIET

If, by this time, you are highly confused about what to eat, it is really quite simple. Just eat whole, natural foods, as many raw as possible.

What will be the results of such a new, whole, natural diet? Good results may not come instantly. At first, one day now and then you will probably feel better until you eventually have more good days than bad. Do not be surprised if you even feel worse at times, in the early days.

You may or may not have fleeting pains, a rash, insomnia, headaches, and other so-called "healing crises." This is because your body chemistry is changing and your body does not like changes. Also toxins may be stirred up and ejected, explaining the rash, for instance. Take it easy, keep it up and sooner or later you will be glad you did! The new and better way you feel will be more than worth any discomfort you experience at first.

It is best not to tell your friends what you are doing. They will chide you and try to dissuade you, as they do when you announce you are going on a reducing diet.

Do your thing in secret and in time they will ask you what you are doing and want to join you. That is time enough to share your secret of good nutrition with them.

NOTES

1. James F. Wallace, M.A., Research Director, and Maureen J. Wallace, Research Analyst, *The Effects of Excessive Consumption of Refined Sugar,* etc. etc., distributed by Parents for Better Nutrition, a non-profit Oregon Corporation, 33 N. Central, Room 200, Medford, OR 97501.
2. Linda Clark, *Stay Young Longer.* New York: Pyramid Publications, 1968. Paperback Edition. Chapter 7: Is Sugar Harmful?
3. Beatrice Trum Hunter, *The Natural Foods Primer.* New York: Simon and Schuster, 1972.

4. Dr. T. L. Cleave, *The Saccharine Disease.* New Canaan, CT: Keats Publishing Co., 1975. Paperback.

5. Susan Smith Jones, *The Main Ingredients: Positive Thinking, Exercise and Diet.* 1978.

6. Barbara Cartland, *The Magic of Honey,* New York: Pyramid Publications, 1973.

7. C. E. Burtis, *Nature's Miracle Medicine Chest,* New York: Arco Publishing Co. Paperback.

8. Dorothy Perlman, *The Magic of Honey.* New York: Avon, 1978.

9. Body Language, a Newsletter, Vol. 3, No. 3, April 1979.

10. Jim Schreiber and Janice Fillip, "Edible Oil: the Cold Facts on Cold Pressed," *Whole Foods* Magazine, 1978.

11. Weston A. Price, D.D.S., *Nutrition and Physical Degeneration.* La Mesa, CA: Price-Pottenger Nutrition Foundation, 1945, 1970.

12. Body Language, a Newsletter, Vol. 3, No. 1, Feb. 1979.

	Mineral Salts	**Water**	**Caloric Value**
Wheat flour	1.0	11.4	1675
Potatoes	1.0	78.3	385
Bananas	.8	75.3	460

These tables show that those who eat whole wheat bread (possibly a superior product for those who can use it) thinking they are saving carbohydrates and calories by avoiding potatoes, are in for a rude shock.

Three-quarters of a cup of mashed potatoes yields only 93 calories, and a medium baked potato only 90 calories, less than the caloric yield of an apple or a pear.

In addition, according to more recent U.S. Dept. of Agriculture reports, potatoes contain some calcium, phosphorus, and the vitamins C, B_1, B_2, folic acid, B_6 and niacin. Potatoes are also, according to these reports, low in sodium, high in potassium and contain iron and magnesium—all minerals.

POTATOES AND WEIGHT LOSS

Although nutritionists and most doctors do not recommend a diet of a single food only, there is one record of a woman weighing 208 pounds who lived mainly on a potato diet for a year (she added some vegetables, eggs, sea foods and fowl as well as yogurt). She lost 83 pounds and was able to wear a size nine dress at the end of the year.

According to the Potato Industry Board, here are two enlightening statements:

"Nature has designed only a few foods that are capable of nourishing the great populations of the world. Of these the white potato is one."

"There are ample reasons why nutritional deficiencies are little known in the countries whose populations depend on potatoes as their basic food."

There are some precautions to observe in the use of potatoes. One guest who has long been a convert to natural foods, and had traveled from New York to California by plane asked me, "What in the world do they do to the mashed potatoes they serve on planes? They taste terrible." The answer: they are processed, not natural.

UNREAL AND REAL

If you will read labels on any boxed or frozen potato product you will find all manner of chemicals and additives present. Reconstituted potatoes, which have been dried and chemicalized are a sad imitation of freshly mashed potatoes, prepared from scratch. One of my greatest pleasures at family holiday dinners is a large pan of creamy, hot, freshly cooked, mashed potatoes prepared by one family member who appreciates, as I do, the natural flavor of freshly prepared potatoes.

Not only does the flavor of potatoes suffer from processing, but the nutritional value as well. Two researchers, one from University of Washington the other from University of Idaho, analyzed the vitamin content at various stages of potato processing. Some of the vitamins were adversely affected by the processing itself, whereas other B vitamins, lying close to the skin, were severely reduced by peeling.

There was vitamin C loss due to blanching (for freezing) as well as later frying which also reduced the level of the vitamin B content.

There are nutrients in or under the potato skin which are advantageous but it is also true that potatoes raised in DDT or other pesticide-treated soils can absorb this poison. For this reason, although I love the skin of a crisply baked potato with its hot fluffy interior, I refuse to eat the skin unless I am sure the potato was grown organically in poison-free soil.

HOW TO AVOID
BAKED POTATO CALORIES

Since many of us believe there is nothing as good as a freshly baked potato, yet do not want to add unnecessary calories from sour cream or extra butter, here are some alternatives:

• For a low calorie topping which tastes as good or better than sour cream, which you can make at home and know that it is safe, (some commercial nondairy imitations, highly promoted, may actually contain twenty-six calories per *tablespoon*) try plain yogurt, which is only eight calories per tablespoonful. And for extra flavor use chopped chives or parsley which add no calories at all. People to whom I have served this topping did not notice the difference from the regular sour cream until I told them.

• Or you can use low fat cottage cheese, plain or whipped, which has only about fifteen calories per tablespoonful. Better yet, try "homemade sour cream" which is made by combining equal parts of cottage cheese and buttermilk or yogurt in your blender. Yield in calories: ten per tablespoonful.

• In order to outwit high calorie gravies and cream sauces to add to your baked or creamed potato, make a cream sauce of one cup skim milk mixed with two tablespoons unbleached flour or two teaspoons arrowroot powder from grocery spice shelves, sea salt, onion flakes and a dash of Worcestershire sauce, all mixed in your blender and stirred constantly on the stove while it is thickening. Less than ten calories per tablespoon.

• Or use the "au jus" or natural juices from a roast and thicken it with flour if you must. You can thicken beef or chicken broth the same way.

The following recipes are from my own cookbook.[2] I must warn you that this cookbook is not necessarily a health cookbook but a collection of my family's treasured recipes, although I have used more healthful ingredients in many of them.

The first recipe is a butter stretcher, considered by some far more healthful as well as cheaper than plain butter. It is good on baked potatoes. The other recipes are for some of my favorite methods of preparing potatoes and I hope you will like them as much as I do.

Meanwhile don't forget about making scalloped potatoes or that wonderful old fashioned potato soup. You will find a recipe for each in almost any cookbook. And if there is any hot potato soup left over, add chicken broth, a dash of Worcestershire sauce, a pinch of nutmeg, and chill to serve cold as vichyssoise. Top with chopped chives. It's great!

So stop feeling guilty about eating potatoes. Use them and enjoy them for the good, nutritious food they are.

BUTTER STRETCHER

1 lb. of butter
1 cup natural vegetable oil (sesame, safflower, or sunflower—from health store)
2-4 tablespoons liquid lecithin (from health stores)

Dissolve the lecithin in the oil in a blender. Let butter soften at room temperature and add the liquid oil–lecithin mixture. Beat all until smooth with an electric beater. (If the liquid lecithin clings to the spoon or inside of the blender, wipe it off with a dry paper towel before washing.)

Store the mixture in covered containers in the refrigerator. It will spread easily on removal from the refrigerator. If you like more salt, add a bit of sea salt before mixing.[2]

QUICK CREAMED POTATOES

Peel and grate five medium sized, raw potatoes into a saucepan. Cover with whole milk or half-and-half. Add 2 tablespoons butter, one grated onion, salt and pepper. Simmer gently, stirring occasionally until potatoes are tender and milk is absorbed, leaving a creamy consistency. Sprinkle with chopped parsley. If the potatoes are finely grated, this recipe will take about ten minutes. Be careful not to scorch! Serves six.

POTATO PANCAKES

Grate four large potatoes and one small onion.
Add:
    ½ cup milk
    1 beaten egg
    2 tablespoons flour
    1 teaspoon salt

Mix and drop by the spoonful on hot griddle, browning on both sides.

Dr. Royal Lee, the late renowned nutrition expert, adds some unusual benefits from potatoes.[3]

He reminds us that Hindhede in Denmark considered the potato protein the finest of all protein for human nutrition. Yet, adds Dr. Lee, potato solids are only ten percent protein. But the potato starch, he says, has an alkaline ash which is far better tolerated than the acid ash from the starch of cereals. Potatoes are easily digested and "supplemented with meat or beans provide a pretty good diet." He believed it is better to eat potatoes than bread. His reasons: they contain many less calories than bread, spaghetti, pies, or cakes. Actually, potatoes are approximately 75% water; 15% starch (of a better type as already explained) and up to two percent protein and close to three percent minerals.

Dr. Lee believes that raw potato is one of the best remedies for constipation. He advocates using thinly sliced raw potato in salads. He says, "The anticonstipation enzyme in potatoes is destroyed by heat. Certainly a piece of raw potato taken before bedtime can do no harm, and it has provided beneficial results in cases of chronic constipation."

Dr. Lee also shares some valuable tips for cooking potatoes:

• Keep cooked potatoes in the refrigerator, or 50% loss of vitamin C can take place in 24 hours; all of it in 72 hours! 90% of the vitamin C can also be lost from mashed potatoes within 30 minutes, if kept hot. So prepare and serve your mashed potatoes at the last minute.

• Cooking potatoes in salt water conserves more vitamin C than cooking in unsalted water.

• Dropping unpeeled potatoes whole into boiling water conserves more nutrients than if you start peeled or whole potatoes cooking in cold water.

• To prevent blackening of raw potato, add one tablespoon vinegar or lemon juice.

• Baked potatoes should be pricked or broken open as soon as they are removed from the oven, to let the steam escape. This prevents sogginess.

• Watch out for potatoes grown where excessive watering is used. This raises the "potato-for-sale weight" but can also reduce the nutrients. A dryer mineral-rich soil, without previous applications of insecticides (which are absorbed by the skins, thus making baked potato skins unacceptable) is preferable.

• Many nutrients lie just beneath the skin, so boil potatoes with the skin, whenever possible.

• Never eat the green potato sprouts. They are considered deadly! Remove them before serving or cooking.

• Avoid using green potatoes.

• Whenever possible grow your own.

If you have any garden space at all, they are easy to grow. I dig a shallow hole (bed); add kelp, wood ashes and bonemeal or garden lime, and drop in store potatoes, cut into pieces, each containing at least one eye.

Cover, water lightly, and harvest when the tall green plants start turning brown.

You can dig or pull them out with your hands and eat skins without worry. They are matchless and delicious.

NOTES

1. Dr. H. Valentine Skaggs, *Potatoes as Food and Medicine.* C. W. Daniel Co., Ltd. Ashington, Rochford, published in Canada by Provoker Press, St. Catharines, Ontario.

2. Linda Clark, *Linda Clark's Cookbook.* San Francisco: Strawberry Hill Press, 1977.

3. *Let's LIVE* Magazine, 1958.

CHAPTER TEN

Is Fiber Really Good for You?

WHAT IS FIBER?

There are various types of fiber. The one we are mainly interested in is dietary fiber, which we can eat and which, in the past few years, has become almost a household word. In many cases the public has grabbed this substance because it promises relief from constipation plus so many approaches to better health that they consider it a cure-all. Is it really a panacea? Let's give fiber an honest appraisal to help you decide if it will *really* help you.

Bran, the best known type of fiber, is the covering of cereal grains and is largely eliminated from grain products by the refining of flour and other whole cereals. It can, however, be added separately to foods to replace the loss.

But bran, as most people forget, is not the only source of fiber. Fruits and vegetables also contain varying amounts of fiber, particularly, as in the case of fruits, when the peeling and seeds are also consumed. For example, apples and pears, eaten with the skins, contribute fiber to the diet. So do berries and nuts of all kinds. Salads, made of raw vegetables, are also an excellent source of fiber.

Dietary fiber, in the form of bran, is not new. It was known as a laxative centuries ago to Hippocrates, considered the "Father of Medicine." Then, in the early 1900s it was extolled in the United States by one of our earliest groups interested in dietetics and nutrition, The Battle Creek (Michigan) Foundation which advocated bran as an aid for constipation.

The next thing to happen was more recent research conducted by several English doctors, particularly Dr. Denis P. Burkitt, an

English surgeon and an internationally known medical researcher. This research showed that African natives had a resistance to bowel cancer, apparently as a result of a high intake of dietary fiber (much higher in fact among these natives on natural foods than our own diet which contains so many refined foods, which eliminate fiber).

Dr. Burkitt and associates showed internal pictures of the intestinal health (or the lack of it) of natives with and without adequate fiber in their diet to doctors internationally. The doctors were stunned and one was heard to remark, "I would not have believed that something you put in your mouth could be so helpful to your health." This is a common reaction with many orthodox practitioners who do not understand nutrition because it is not taught in the average medical school.

As a result of this conversion through exposure to the pictures, doctors began to take fiber themselves and prescribe it for their patients. Now, since the earlier research on the role of fiber in preventing bowel cancer, Dr. Burkitt has done further research and learned that fiber can also help *prevent* other body ailments, namely: appendicitis, diabetes, excess cholesterol, diverticulitis, gall stones, hiatal hernia, hemorrhoids, varicose veins and other disturbances. Fiber, because it is low in calories has also been found to play a part in weight control. But unfortunately, the public has seized upon fiber as a panacea, elevating it to a sweeping fad. Products on the grocery shelves now scream: "This product contains fiber!" to entice gullible buyers. And although research does stand behind the statement that fiber can be helpful in many conditions, it has since been found that *for some people* and *some conditions* it can also be dangerous.

So let's separate facts from fancies.

DANGERS OF FIBER

Barbara Kraus, in her book, *Guide to Fiber in Foods,*[1] says, "There is danger to some individuals in radically increasing the amount of fibrous foods in their diets. They should follow the dietary recommendations of their physicians.

"Fiber is not a cure-all for all the ills of our society, but is mainly for the average healthy person," she warns.

On the other hand, in some instances where fibrous foods have been previously banned by physicians from the diets of those suffering from diverticulitis, the use of fiber has actually been found by Dr. Burkitt and his associates to be most helpful for this condition. So doctors as well as patients should do their homework on the subject of fiber.

Dr. Harold Harper, biochemist and nutrition professor of the University of California School of Medicine, warns that high fiber diets may be potentially dangerous for some people. He says that too much fiber can increase attacks of colitis or cause diarrhea in some people. He adds that when pain and cramping occur, "The worst possible thing is a high fiber diet."[2]

I have known some people and one Great Dane dog who had rectal bleeding after taking bran, perhaps because of an irritable colon, or a sensitive stomach or intestinal lining. I asked the people and the dog owner if this were due to an especially high roughage content in some brans they used. The answer was no, that they used the refined health store type bran, because it was softer and "less scratchy."

WATCH OUT FOR PHYTIN

Another problem with bran is that it is high in phytin, a substance which prevents the body's proper assimilation of calcium, iron, zinc, copper and magnesium.[3] There is a solution to this problem. If you soak your dry bran in water overnight or even up to twenty-four hours, before using it, the antagonism to these minerals is lessened. Yeast and acid added to bran foods before cooking also help to break down phytin. But once bran (untreated) is cooked, it is too late to change the phytin content.

Some people who are wheat intolerant can use bran; others can't. So you have to feel your own way in using bran. We will discuss how much is best shortly.

OTHER TYPES OF FIBER

One of the greatest problems in the fiber craze is the substitution of powdered wood cellulose (sawdust) to commercially made breads.

Read your labels; if the fiber is bran, it should say *Bran.* If it is wood fiber, the term used is "cellulose." Tests are not yet available to ascertain if this wood cellulose is dangerous to humans or not. Controversy on the subject exists. Some claim that fiber is fiber; others, including Dr. Harper, believe that the use of wood cellulose (sawdust) in food borders on the fraudulent.[2]

Still another type of fiber, called *crude fiber,* often found in prepared cereals, is the indigestible factor from certain plants which remains even after rigorous chemical treatment. Crude fiber is allowed in some breads as well as cereals. Again, the best way to go is to read the labels which should indicate the type of fiber added to foodstuffs. Those who know they are wheat intolerant may wish to substitute rice bran for wheat. Rice bran is available in most health stores and some regular groceries.

Beatrice Trum Hunter in her book, *The Great Nutrition Robbery*[3] adds her concern about the possible excessive use of fiber. She is also concerned with the type of fiber you use. She describes the wood cellulose problem in detail, and she is an honest researcher, who can be trusted to tell you the truth.

In addition to the need for pretreating the phytin in bran, most nutritionists believe that fiber is important to health, particularly if it is used in the form of vegetables, and fruits in moderation. Meanwhile, to avoid the use of excessive fiber you need to learn how much fiber is effective as well as safe for you. There are clues to help you.

HOW MUCH FIBER IS BEST FOR YOU?

No one has actually determined the amount of fiber to be used. This, no doubt, is due to individual needs and differences. Most nutritionists feel that a well balanced diet which includes leafy vegetables, legumes and fruit, and whole grain bread and cereals, (*if you are not intolerant to them*) provide an adequate supply of fiber. Raw salads help you here, too.

Those who can tolerate bran, should, according to Dr. Carlton Fredericks, start with a teaspoonful a day, whereas others may need three tablespoons daily.[4] If your stool is easy, comfortable to eject, full and firm, you are apparently using the right amount for you, he believes. If, on the other hand your stool is like small pebbles or hard and dry, you may need more fiber. Also, bran absorbs six times its weight in water, making a softer stool easier to eliminate. So for best results be sure to drink plenty of water when taking bran.[1]

Diarrhea or an over-laxative effect may mean you are taking too much fiber. As Dr. Fredericks writes, "When your stool is largely free of odor, formed well, large in amount, and requires no strain in evacuation, the right level of bran intake has been established."

HOW TO CHOOSE FIBER FOODS

If you buy fiber-fortified cereals and breads, read your labels to learn whether that fiber is bran, wood cellulose (sawdust) or crude fiber. In my opinion, the label should also tell you how much bran is included in each slice of bread, muffin or one-half cup serving of cereal. This should not be too difficult for the manufacturers to compute. They could take the amount approximately contained in a loaf of bread, count the slices and come up with the amount of bran contained in one slice.

Then you would know how much you are getting, whether it is too much or if you should add more to your diet.

The best way of all to be sure you are using bran or other grains safely in bread, muffins, or as cereals is to prepare your own. The following recipe is one I have evolved over a period of time, and which is popular. People who make these bran muffins write me that they love them, and at least one health store serves them at its food counter.

Here is a recipe to get you started. Experiment from time to time until you are happy with results.

BRAN MUFFINS

To eliminate phytic acid, soak overnight (eight hours or as long as twenty-four hours if desired): two cups of bran flakes (from health store) in four cups of cool water. When ready to mix the muffins, drain off the water, which is rich in minerals, reserving it to add to soups, sauces, juices or pet food. It can also be used to fertilize your plants. (It does not contain phytic acid.)

Mix the other liquids, including an egg, 1 cup of milk or buttermilk, honey to taste (about 3 tablespoons) and 3 tablespoons of oil and 1 tablespoon of bakers' yeast, which has been dissolved in 1 cup warm water. Mix all liquids in a blender.

In a bowl mix dry ingredients, using 1 cup flour (whole wheat or unbleached), a pinch of salt, 3 teaspoons of baking powder (health store).

Add liquids to dry ingredients and stir gently. (Never beat muffin batter). For flavoring, add 1 cup fresh or unsweetened frozen blueberries, or chopped apple, whole raisins or reconstituted, cut dried apricots. If using apples or raisins, also add the spices which you prefer, approximately 1 heaping teaspoon cinnamon and 1/8 teaspoon *each* of allspice, ground cloves and nutmeg. Stir in, mixing gently. (1 cup of nut meats or sunflower seeds, or a mixture of both is optional.) Now add the drained, soaked bran a little at a time, mixing it with the other ingredients until you have a thick batter which drops, not flows from a spoon. If you have used yeast allow the batter to rise at room temperature until double before baking.

Fill oiled muffin tins half full and bake at 400° until firm and lightly browned on top. Makes twelve or more muffins. Any leftover batter, if made with yeast or double acting baking powder, can be refrigerated and then baked the second day. Any leftover muffins can be sliced and toasted for next day's breakfast. Any soaked bran that isn't used in the muffins can be saved to add to cereal, cookies, meatloaf or other foods if you need more fiber.

WHERE TO OBTAIN FIBER

To get more natural fiber into your diet, grow your own food if possible. Sprouted seeds are an excellent source of fiber. Organically grown apples, peaches, plums, apricots, pears and berries provide fiber if the skin and, if possible, seeds are eaten. Vegetables providing fiber include potatoes (eat the skins only if organically raised), carrots (preferably scrubbed but unpeeled), cabbage, cauliflower, brussels sprouts, broccoli, beans, celery, peppers, cucumbers with seeds, summer squash and zucchini, plus corn, asparagus, peas, edible pod peas, even some wild herbs like Lamb's Quarters—the sky is the limit. Vegetables should be eaten raw or undercooked (slightly steamed or stir-fried, Oriental style).

And remember, at least one raw salad per day.

Following is an excellent article written by Emory Thurston, containing more information on the importance and use of fiber:

THE IMPORTANCE OF FIBER*

Emory W. Thurston, Ph.D., Sc.D.

Since the publication of Dr. Denis P. Burkitt's research on the relationship of fiber in the diet to the health of the colon, the importance of dietary fiber has been a much discussed topic in nutrition circles and in the news media. Whole books have been written on the subject. From the publicity, one might think that fiber is a new discovery. Listen to Hippocrates in 430 B.C. "You people, complaining of your health, should pass large, bulky motions after every meal, and that to insure this, you should eat abundantly of whole meal bread, vegetables and fruits . . ."

Heretofore the word "roughage" has generally been used when speaking of this essential adjunct to the diet, and it has been more or less assumed that the fruits and vegetables in the diet would provide a sufficient amount. The great increase in constipation and diseases of the colon since the turn of the century attests that no such assumption was justified. The number of deaths from colon cancer is second only to that of lung cancer, and it is estimated that a large percentage of the people in this country suffer with various diseases of the colon—frequently forerunners of cancer. Among such disorders are polyps, ulcerative colitis, spastic colon, appendicitis, hemorrhoids, and diverticulitis (inflammation of abnormal "pockets" in the muscular lining

*Reprinted by permission from *PPNF Bulletin* Vol. 1 No. 3, September 1976.

of the colon). Dr. Burkitt's work with people of different cultures has shown that none of these diseases occurs when high-residue diets are eaten. *Such a diet contains 25-30 grams of fiber daily.* It is said that the average diet in this country has less than 5 grams.

My experience in analyzing diets reveals that even nutrition-conscious people often have much less than 5 grams. Those who think they eat a good breakfast—perhaps juice, eggs and breakfast meat, one slice of toast (usually white or so-called whole wheat), and a beverage—receive practically no fiber in such a meal. If the toast were 100 percent whole wheat, the fiber content of the meal would be boosted to almost 0.3 grams! If the juice were replaced with a whole fruit such as an apple, orange, banana, or half of a large grapefruit, approximately one gram would be added. What about lunch for a person who is attempting to eat properly? It may include a green salad (often only two large green leaves of lettuce—0.2 grams of fiber, and one medium tomato—0.6 grams), one slice whole wheat bread—0.3 grams, and whatever else is eaten for protein, salad dressing, dessert, and beverage, none of which will add to the fiber content—unless the dessert is fruit. Midday snacks are not likely to consist of fiber foods, so by dinner time our nutrition-minded friend has had all of 1.1 grams of fiber, unless we count the suggested breakfast substitutions, which would increase the total fiber intake to 2.4 grams [instead of the suggested 25 grams.]

Surely he will make up the remaining twenty odd grams at dinner; let us see. Besides the meat, fish or fowl protein entree (no fiber) we will include a grated carrot salad (½ cup carrots—0.6 grams of fiber, and 2 tablespoonfuls raisins—0.2 grams), ½ cup potato—0.3 grams, and ½ cup summer squash—0.3 grams. Adding this 1.4 grams of dinner fiber to the 2.4 grams taken at breakfast and lunch we have a total for the day of 3.8 grams! Let us be good to our friend and give him a nutritious high-fiber dinner dessert or evening snack of one cup of strawberries—1.9 grams of fiber. This brings the total for the day to 5.7 grams—slightly over the 5 grams which is claimed to be the average for the country, *not* the 25-30 needed. The amount of fruits, vegetables, and whole grains in this menu is far more than the average person has in a day. Furthermore, this menu is especially favored by the inclusion of apple or banana, lettuce and carrot—all sources of a particularly useful type of fiber. More about this later.

Just think of the many people who have for breakfast only juice, coffee, and a cigarette—perhaps a donut or sweetroll (no fiber), or even a cup of cornflakes—0.1 grams of fiber. (One fourth cup of crude bran would provide almost fourteen times that amount.) Lunch might be any of these fiberless foods: soup, sandwich, hamburger, hot dog, pie or other such dessert. A "good" dinner might consist of meat, potato, gravy, a serving of cooked vegetable, and a salad. It would be very easy for one to think he is eating a "well-balanced" diet and at the same time have practically no fiber. The day's menu just described would provide, at the most, only 3 to 4 grams of fiber. There is little wonder that the laxative business flourishes as it does in this country.

How did we get into such a state? Several factors have contributed. Before the beginning of this century practically all breads and cereals were whole grain, and much more of them were eaten. The more physically active life of our ancestors was to their advantage in at least two ways. In the natural course of their activities they had the exercise which most of us must contrive to have and often fail to achieve, and they needed and could metabolize twice as many calories as we can. Not only do we eat less whole grains than formerly, but also less fruits and vegetables. At the same time our consumption of fats, sugars, and refined, processed foods of all kinds has increased so that many people take more calories than they need and suffer the consequences in various ways.

The spin-off of this situation has led not only to the increase of colon disease, but also to such complications as heart disease, diabetes, obesity, and varicose veins. Dr. Burkitt found that this same fate befalls the rural African when he leaves his native area and his high-residue diet containing some 25 grams of fiber, and moves to the city where he adopts the European diet with probably not more than 5 grams of fiber. It is not long before he begins to suffer the complaints of "civilization," all unknown in his native habitat. Undoubtedly other factors in his new life-style contribute to this degeneration in his health. The stress of urban living and probably having much less sunshine and exercise than he is accustomed to, as well as other differences, would all have an effect on his well-being.

In our overfed and undernourished population, choosing a dietary to provide sufficient fiber is somewhat of a problem, as was seen in the example of the day's menu discussed earlier. (The figures given in that menu are only approximate, being averages of the widely varying figures found in several tables giving the crude fiber content of foods.) Whole, natural health-food-store bran is generally considered to be the best fiber food because it absorbs water and tends to produce soft, bulky stools. It also is resistant to bacterial attack, which may break down other types of plant fiber.

Since bran absorbs seven to eight times its weight in water, it is important that sufficient liquid be taken with it so as not to draw water from the body tissues. For this reason [as well as for removing phytin] it should be soaked overnight, or at least for some time before it is eaten. If the schedule allows, it is probably better to take portions with each meal instead of all at one time.

The amount taken depends upon the individual situation. This would be none at all for people afflicted with certain colon problems. Others might start with two teaspoonfuls each meal and gradually increase if needed. Some take as much as two or three tablespoonsful three times a day. Small amounts can be sneaked into all sorts of foods, but this would not suffice for one who is in need of a therapeutic dose. There are tastier foods which can be eaten with bran to "help the medicine go down!" For example, fruit (try grated apple—or any other fruit) and cottage cheese or yogurt, or mix with another more savory cereal (oatmeal, cornmeal, or other whole meal), or wheat germ—if you have access to it weekly just after milling when it is absolutely fresh. Rancid oils are dangerous. The germ of the wheat is the source of wheat germ oil, so also beware of rancid wheat germ. Freshly milled wheat germ is sweet, but the flavor deteriorates rapidly and becomes bitter.

Since the phosphorus content of both bran and wheat germ is so much higher than that of calcium, and since it is important to keep the ratio of these two elements in balance, calcium lactate or gluconate should be added when these foods are taken. When calcium is added, magnesium also should be added.

Other sources of fiber are ground or well-chewed whole grains, nuts, and seeds (sunflower, pumpkin, sesame, flax, alfalfa). Besides fiber, these foods also supply natural oils. The amount of these foods eaten will, to some extent, depend upon the calories one can "afford."

Millet and rolled oats are good grain fiber foods, as well as being excellent sources of other nutrients. It has long been my custom to have rolled oats frequently. Soak overnight, cook slightly, and for extra nutrition and complete protein stir in one or two eggs per person at the last minute. Or have the eggs separately, and flavor the oats with any kind of dried fruit—raisins, dates, prunes, apricots, figs, peaches, pears—which will also add fiber.

Raw or slightly cooked starch presents a digestive problem for some people. In these cases grains should be cooked longer. Possibly this problem would be solved by longer chewing rather than by longer cooking, since starches must be well mixed with saliva for complete digestion. Another reason for difficulty in digesting cereals is the addition of sugar and milk or cream. If fruits are not used and sweetening is needed, a small amount of honey or lactose should be used—never sugar. Try eating cereals without milk or cream. Cottage cheese and yogurt are less likely to cause digestive upset and combine well with fruit and cereal.

Good fiber "buys" in vegetables are celery and the leafy greens (beet tops, broccoli, cabbage, chard, lettuce, spinach). How often and how much of these are eaten by the general population? Among other vegetables with relatively high fiber for the calories carried are artichoke, asparagus, green beans, green peas, parsnips, summer and winter squash, and tomatoes. All dried beans, peas, and lentils are high in fiber but also high in calories. Root vegetables are good fiber foods.

Fruits are higher than vegetables in the calories they carry for the fiber they contain. The best "buys" are blackberries, strawberries, cantaloupes, watermelon, papaya, grapefruit, oranges, apples, and bananas. Actually, because of the type of fiber they contain, apples and bananas are two of the best fiber foods.

Foods have various types of fiber—cellulose, hemicellulose, lignin, pectin—which differ in their digestibility as well as end products. As much as 50 percent of the fiber of fruits and vegetables may be digested and therefore not available as roughage. Those foods with the most lignin, a type of fiber highly resistant to digestion, may be considered, along with bran, to be the best fiber foods. Among these are bananas, apples, lettuce, carrots, and cabbage. Lignin does not increase the bulk of the stool as does the hemicellulose of bran, whole grains, and some other foods, but in some way, not yet fully understood, it assists in the digestive process.

Another variable in the matter of fiber is that individuals differ in their handling of the various fibers in the intestine. In some people bacteria are present which decompose the fiber so that it fails in its function to stimulate evacuation. This can account for some cases of constipation even when large amounts of fruits and vegetables are eaten. These individuals, unless they have some disease of the colon, probably need bran, which resists such bacterial action.

Bran and other roughage are not recommended for those with intestinal adhesions or stenosis (narrowing of the intestine). Some physicians, however, have successfully reversed their treatment of diverticulitis from a soft, low-residue diet to one which includes fiber foods. Those not in the habit of eating fiber foods would be wise to eat sparingly of them at first, gradually increasing the amount. Bananas are a good transition food, as they are high in fiber but less irritating than other fiber foods. Cooked rather than raw fruits and vegetables also are less irritating while still providing bulk. [Some people are intolerant of some foods, including citrus fruits and bananas.]

In cases where the colon cannot tolerate excessive roughage, the edible mucilaginous substances known as hydrophilic colloids are useful. Some of the sources of these are psyllium seed, flax seed, karaya, guar, Irish moss, and other sea plants—the sources of carrageen and agar-agar. As with bran, these substances absorb many times their weight in water producing a smooth bulk to stimulate peristalsis. Read labels when buying these products. A drug store brand, which is sold more than any other, is fifty percent sugar (dextrose). Selling at over $4.00 for 14 ounces, this is expensive sugar, besides being one of the causes of the ailment for which the product is needed! Another drug store brand is sugar-free, and two other sugar-free brands are available at some health food stores and from some chiropractors. One brand, sold mostly by chiropractors, is forty percent sugar, although the label does not reveal this important information.

Pectins, although classified as hemicellulose, behave more like colloids because of their capacity to absorb water. The mention of pectin probably brings to mind apples. The pectin and lignin content of this fruit are two more reasons for the validity of the old adage: An apple a day keeps the doctor away.

Among the first solid carbohydrate foods recommended for babies are scraped apple and banana. Later, when their molar teeth appear they are ready for the complex carbohydrates. At that time properly prepared whole grains (not a commercial substitute) should be a part of the daily intake. A diet supplying a liberal amount of fruits, vegetables, nuts, seeds, and the whole grains and with no refined carbohydrates will do much to ensure a healthy colon throughout life.

Many "new discoveries" in nutrition are popularized and eagerly accepted by an ailing public looking for panaceas. Dietary fiber is as important as Hippocrates knew it to be and as it was long before his time. But to be completely effective, other basic health principles must not be neglected—particularly exercise. All factors are interdependent for optimum health.

At the end of a day in which your intake of fiber is low you may use a prepared fiber mixture. One type is called *Fy-Blend,* available at health stores. Another is Veico's *Intestinal Cleanser,* available from Price Pottenger Nutrition Foundation.

In either case, stir 1 tablespoon of the mixture into water and drink quickly. You may take just before bedtime or night and morning if necessary. Either should give you good intestinal elimination, according to the reports of those who have used this type of product.

The following excerpt from the November, 1979 issue of the newsletter, *Body Language* offers some worthy advice.

TO ENRICH YOUR DIET WITH FIBER:

- serve raspberries or blackberries
- sprinkle crushed bran on baked potato
- add chopped unpeeled apples or green pepper to cottage cheese
- use bran for breading meat or poultry
- add sunflower seeds to sandwich mixes and salads
- add chopped dates to cream cheese
- eat raw fruits for dessert

NOTES

1. Barbara Kraus, *The Guide to Fiber in Food.* New York: New American Library, 1975.

2. Judith Anderson, "The Food Fad of the Year," San Francisco *Chronicle,* July 6, 1977.

3. Beatrice Trum Hunter, *The Great Nutrition Robbery.* New York: Scribners, 1978 (and other medical references by personal communication).

4. Carlton Fredericks, Ph.D., *Dr. Carlton Fredericks' New and Complete Nutrition Handbook: Your Key to Good Health,* Chatsworth, CA: Major Books, 1978.

CHAPTER ELEVEN

Some Nutritional Miracles

Obviously nutrition is not going to be a cure-all for everyone, particularly when the cause of an ailment is due to something else, such as unsolved psychological problems, heredity, exposure to poisons and contaminated environment, etc. Still, even these may be lessened by the adoption of an overall nutritious diet such as we have been describing, thus giving the body better nervous control, immunity and resistance, plus added energy, in addition to correcting a deficiency which may be the source of the problem.

There are many orthodox therapists who do not understand nutrition, and when drugs (which are usually temporary in effect) do not bring success, they give up too easily by advising the patient to see a psychiatrist; or tell the patient that nothing can be done for her ailment but to learn to live with it. This does not mean that a psychiatrist cannot be helpful, if the need is really there, but many people have heard this verdict only because the original doctor did not know what else to do and therefore swept all unsolved problems into the psychiatric or you'll-have-to-learn-to-live-with-it wastebasket. There are millions of people who after such a discouraging diagnosis still received help from nutrition and became completely well. So don't give up until you have tried nutrition, too.

SAVING MARRIAGES

Good nutrition has even saved marriages. Cecilia Rosenfeld, M.D., a nutrition-oriented physician as well as general practitioner, has long used nutrition to repair marriages. So has the North Nassau Mental Health Center, Manhasset, NY. According to Dr. David Hawkins, psychiatrist and medical director of this Center, in one year alone, of the ninety percent of the couples who came for marriage counseling, forty-five percent had a nutritional disorder which had caused the marital difficulties.[1]

Dr. Hawkins admitted that inadequate nutrition is often the cause of marital discord, or at least an aggravating factor.[1] This pronouncement, please notice, came from a *psychiatrist.*

Mary Jane Hungerford, Ph.D., a nutritional consultant and director of the American Institute of Family Relations in Santa Barbara, California, agrees. She finds that most of the problems which appear at this institute can also be traced to malnutrition as a result of a lifelong habit of eating white sugar and flour, plus inadequate protein. Fatigue plays a big role in this, she says. The couples use candy, cigarettes or alcohol as a crutch.[1] Often they are suffering from hypoglycemia, in which case even a cup of coffee can trigger an outburst of anger.

Dr. Hawkins cites the example of a typical hypoglycemic couple. The wife was eating candy and drinking soda pop for energy pickups. She was overweight. Her husband had acquired a girl friend, and he was drinking alcohol. Both wanted a divorce. When they were taken off of sweets and alcohol, and given a nutritional program, their behavior approached normal and eight years later, they were still doing fine.[1]

NUTRITION FOR VIOLENCE AND CRIME

It is common knowledge now that hyperactive children often respond favorably to the removal of synthetic additives from the diet, a concept advocated by Ben F. Feingold, M.D. However, it may not be as well known that there is agreement in many high places that violence and crime can also result from poor diet in both children and adults.

One researcher to note the correlation between crime and inadequate nutrition is Alexander D. Schauss, Correction Training Officer, Washington State Criminal Justice Training Commission. As a youth in Hamburg, Germany, Schauss noted that Hitler was addicted to chocolate sweets, therefore presumably a hypoglycemic.

Now involved in criminal rehabilitation work, Schauss urges a "sound mind in a sound body" and has found that nutrition is one of the greatest factors in criminal rehabilitation. He advocates good food, and supplements, even hair tests for mineral deficiencies as well as consistent physical exercise, no matter what season of the year.[3]

Barbara Reed, a probation officer for fifteen years, from Cuyahoga Falls, Ohio, has also received national publicity for her use of nutrition in an anti-crime diet. Due to her influence and insistence upon nutritional testing (hypoglycemia was found to be a major factor) she says not one of the cited two hundred and fifty-two persons were returned to court for trouble if they stayed on their improved nutritional program.[4]

Barbara Reed, Alex Schauss, and Dr. Leonard Hippchen, associate professor of the Department of Justice and Public Safety, Virginia Commonwealth University and author of the book, *The Ecologic-Biochemical Approaches to the Treatment of Delinquents and Criminals*[5] states that the nutritional approaches to the rehabilitation of criminals is both new and has an astounding success rate. Alex Schauss predicts that within ten years the nutritional therapy concept will be accepted in all correctional programs.[4]

A hidden food allergy in milk has also been found to be a possible cause of crime.[4] In analyzing diets of criminals and delinquents, researchers state that many of the offenders drank tremendous amounts of milk. Some of the diets discovered are incredible:[4]

From a 10 year old arsonist:
- Breakfast: pre-sweetened cereals, plus equal amounts of milk and soda pop.

From a 16 year old offender:
- Lunch: soda pop, milk, beer and a marijuana joint.
- Bedtime Snack: ice cream; beer, milk and another marijuana joint.

From a 17 year old auto thief:
- Dinner: large amounts of milk and fried chicken; nothing else—no fruits, vegetables, salads or raw food

According to Barbara Reed and Alex Schauss, today *more than one million children and adults are already on probation in the U.S.*[4]

Malnourished people, as well as hypoglycemics, when questioned following their crime, even murder, often admit they did not know why they did it. Later investigations revealed violent rages or depression. Auto accidents are common. Some train motormen have crashed their trains through barricades, also without knowing why. Their characteristic explanations include, "everything went black," or "my head felt funny" or "there was a roaring in my ears." All of these reactions are not uncommon in hypoglycemia, the result of junk food, sweets and other fractionated foods, actually, a completely fractionated *diet!* So, correct nutrition can prevent or correct criminal behavior.

OTHER NUTRITIONAL MIRACLES

Success stories also abound for so-called normal people (if there is such a creature, considering the many individual differences, and anatomical and genetic variations).

One young woman is an impressive example. She was serving as a full time counselor and therapist for family service agencies, was in the midst of preparing her dissertation as a Ph.D. candidate and involved in various other types of research. She found herself becoming increasingly depressed and her husband, a psychologist and full time employee at a private psychiatric institute, suggested that she visit a nutrition consultant as well as a nutritionally oriented doctor, to have her diet checked. Both practitioners recommended that she read a book on hypoglycemia. She then realized that she had, in her busy schedule, been shortchanging herself diet-wise and had been sometimes subsisting on too many carbohydrates, or eating only toast and coffee for breakfast. After adding the suggested supplements, she said, "I never remember feeling better. I feel more full of energy than I ever thought possible.'' She completed her dissertation and is now a full fledged Ph.D. as well as a reformed ''nutritional cripple.''[6]

John Diamond, M.D., the expert in muscle testing, tells of the improvement due to better nutrition in twin girls. These children suffered from stomach cramps, and Dr. Diamond said their behavior was a disaster. They raced noisily around his office, knocking things over and acting like perfect nuisances. He muscle-tested them and showed how sugar could make them weak, but organic, unsprayed apples could make them strong. They were willing to change their diet, and give up their junk food additives, plus any form of processed sugar.

Two weeks later they returned, calm, quiet, well-behaved and polite. The stomach cramps had disappeared. At school they had apparently showed their classmates through muscle testing the bad effect of sugar. As a result their classmates were now trying to swap their junk food for the twins' apples.[7]

ANSWERS TO QUESTIONS FROM READERS

(NOTE: the following questions were chosen because they are representative of the most frequently requested information. Since I am not a doctor, I am, of course, not legally allowed to diagnose, prescribe or suggest).

Q.   When you recommend whole foods, does this mean to eat the skins of fruits, potatoes, and other foods?

A.   Only if these foods have not come in contact with sprays, or other poisons. For example, if fruit such as apples have been sprayed you will often find the residue collected at the base of the stem. Peel before eating. It may be harmless, but is more likely to be poisonous. Potatoes, like fruits, have many nutrients directly under the skin, but if they are grown in soil which has been treated with pesticides, fungicides, or chemical fertilizers, it is safer *not* to eat the skin, including that of a baked potato.

If buying apples or cucumbers, some of which are waxed or coated with mineral oil to look more tempting and sell better, avoid the skin. Peel before eating.

Lettuce and American artichokes are often sprayed with pesticides by helicopters as they grow in the fields. The pesticide collects in the crevices and folds and cannot be washed away. If the poison is already in the soil, it is taken up by the plant roots in growing and also cannot be washed away.

Strawberries, at least those commercially grown in California are often sprayed with arsenic, a fact which the growers have admitted to me. These berries may be sold throughout the United States. If I cannot raise my own produce which has not been treated with such poisonous pesticides, I search for an honest grower who does not use them. Some red potatoes are not really red, but dyed with questionable red coloring. Watch out for other tricks and tampered-with foods! You can even be fooled by produce displayed under hidden, colored lights, which makes the produce look greener and riper than it really is. Our goal is to buy and eat food which is really natural, not that which is made to look natural when it isn't.[8]

HOW TO EAT WELL ON LESS MONEY

Q.   We who are elderly need help. I am over 75, tired and arthritic. I admit to having been a bad eater. But doctors do not seem to even want to talk to us old folks with our aged and worn-out bodies. I would like to eat better but food is high and vitamins out of sight. I am a loner living on social security. I live in a fourteen story building, beside a seventeen story building, both of which include elderly citizens, a few men, and more women. We are all trying to live better but need more information. We need someone to answer our questions to help us eat right.

A.   You are not forgotten. I have written a book about the problems of the elderly and how to rehabilitate yourself. It is called *Rejuvenation.*[9] I also write a Q.A. column, called, "Extend Your Lifeline" which is available in a newsletter called *Good Health Keeping,* published by a nutrition group. You can write to *Good Health Keeping,* P.O. Box 2614, La Mesa, California 92041, and ask about subscription prices. You could join others in subscribing so the cost for each would be less expensive per person. And you may ask as many questions as you like, free. Meanwhile I will start you off with some help on how to get more for your food money.

1. Learn to choose and prepare good food cheaply.

a. Choose foods which are combinations of several nutrients, rather than containing one element alone. These give you more for the money and are cheaper in the long run. They include the so-called power foods, or wonder foods such as brewer's yeast, wheat germ, sunflower seeds, blackstrap molasses and others. A little of each of these foods goes a long way as each one is loaded with many nutrients, rather than just one.

b. For the same reason, use whole, not fractionated foods whenever possible. Use, for example, whole brown rice (delicious) instead of white rice. Whole brown rice contains B vitamins in the outer layer, called rice polishings. These same rice polishings are taken off the whole rice and sold as B vitamins at a higher price, leaving the remaining white rice less nutritious. Use also, if you are not intolerant to them, whole grains, such as wheat, barley, rye, and corn meal which has not been degerminated, (a process which removes the vitamin E for which you will pay dearly if purchased separately). Whenever possible use the whole grains in making your own bread. Buy whole nuts, preferably in the shell, and eat them uncooked for added enzymes. Shelled nuts are now sky high in price. Get the whole nuts through your co-op and shell your own. Raw sunflower seeds, previously mentioned are excellent, a nutritious snack, with many nutrients present plus many health benefits.

c. Ferment your own foods, such as sauerkraut, kosher dill pickles, fermented milks including yogurt, Piima, and cottage cheese; and make your own sourdough bread and rolls which are beneficial even though cooked. (All fermented foods are predigested. In cooked foods the ferments have done their predigesting work before cooking.)

d. Eat as many foods as possible raw. If your teeth can't take them, buy, perhaps jointly, a juicer, and drink the raw juice immediately before enzyme loss takes place. Nutritionists recommend that at least fifty percent of your diet be raw.

e. If you have a garden surplus, purchase a food dryer, jointly. Such foods do not need jars (plastic bags, only) and are more healthful than canned food for winter storage. You may reconstitute them in water before light cooking, or eat as is. A dryer eventually pays for itself.

f. Cod-liver oil has produced many benefits, according to Dale Alexander, in his book, *Arthritis and Common Sense,* and Dr. Price in his book *Nutrition and Physical Degeneration,* which tells of healings from whole foods and grains and cod-liver oil.

If you loathe cod-liver oil (as I do) it can still be palatable. Reserve a small empty jar for no other use and do not wash with your dishes, (the odor is penetrating). To clean the jar, wipe out with a dry paper towel, then if you must, wash separately in a natural detergent and water.

Buy Norwegian cod-liver oil, presumably less processed, and higher in vitamins A, D, and E. Get the mint flavor and keep it refrigerated. In the small jar each morning put about two tablespoons of cold fruit juice, either fresh squeezed natural orange, grape or apple juice, (not additive-filled imitations) and pour over it about a tablespoon of cod-liver oil. Put the lid on the jar, shake well and drink directly from the jar. This should be taken on an empty stomach. If the ingredients are cold from the refrigerator, you will find this a delightful mixture, even if you thought you hated the stuff. The first improvements you will notice are a new sheen on your hair and skin within a week or two. Other results, sometimes relief from arthritis, may take several months, as they come gradually. If you have any doubts, read Dale Alexander's book on arthritis and cod-liver oil which is now published in many countries, many languages.

g. Make your own sprouts and use them in raw salads (do not cook!) or combine several kinds of raw cereal using wheat, barley, rye, mung beans or any mixture you wish, for breakfast, adding a dollop of honey and whole, not skim milk—raw, if you can get it. Dr. Edward Howell, the enzyme researcher, believes that sprouts are the best rejuvenating foods available.

There are many ways to make sprouts; you do not need fancy gadgets. My favorite, and cheapest method is to use a kitchen colander and some white paper towels. Soak the seeds overnight (from health stores *not those coated with dangerous pesticides or fungicides from nursery suppliers!*). In the morning remove the water (use it to water your house plants) and put a layer of seeds on top of a paper towel inside the bottom of the colander. Cover with another towel and add another layer of seeds. Top with a paper towel. Now gently moisten the towels and seeds. Drain and put it in the corner of your kitchen counter and forget until the next morning. Water again daily until the seeds have developed tails about the length of the seeds (except for mung beans, which are longer like the ones you see in the stores). When sprouted, rinse and store in a plastic bag in the refrigerator until needed.

By this time the vitamin and mineral nutrients have skyrocketed to phenomenal levels, as tested in laboratories, yielding free vitamins and minerals for you!

h. For extra vitamin C you may have to buy ascorbic acid, as it is called and is one of the most common factors of the vitamin C family. It is inexpensive. For the remaining factors, called bioflavonoids, a name for the whole C family, you can peel that orange from which you used the juice for cod liver oil and eat the white membrane just under the skin! Far cheaper than what you buy. You are also using the *whole orange,* another unfractionated food.

i. Eggs are still one of our best buys and are considered the Number One Protein used as a standard of measurement for all other proteins. Fertlizied or fertile eggs are far more nutritious, despite any propaganda to the contrary. Why? Fertile eggs hatch, infertile eggs do not. The fertile eggs must contain the extra nutrients to help build life into the tiny chicks. Fertile eggs depend on a rooster and hens should run on the ground, not sit in wire cages, to be healthy, or lay healthful eggs. Use eggs any way you wish but the soft boiled are hard to beat, nutrition-wise. The yolk should still be soft or liquid, thus closer to natural.

j. A green drink is both delicious as well as a powerhouse of nutrients.

RECIPE FOR GREEN DRINK

1 cup of juice (unsweetened pineapple is excellent for flavor) plus 1 cup water. But into a blender and add a handful of any natural

healthful green leaves available. Comfrey and mint are excellent. Blend until the fiber is liquified. If you wish protein, add a handful of sunflower seeds. Pour into a glass over ice cubes (made of juice if you wish) and enjoy!

If you do not have comfrey or mint outdoors, grow them in flower pots on your window sills. Coffee cans with soil will do as well. Parsley and chives and other herbs can also be grown indoors this way, free except for the price of the seeds. Comfrey and mint leaves can also be used as herb teas.

k. *Eat a raw apple a day*

That "apple a day keeps the doctor away" is no joke. We are learning that pectin found in apples is a body detoxifier. One woman I know eats one at bedtime and is still healthy at eighty. And when you shop, READ LABELS. Avoid chemicals and additives whenever possible.

2. I suggest that you start others reading about nutrition so you will all understand the same approach. Some people may not know the truth about additives and pesticides, and other problems in today's food. To do this you could pool your money to jointly buy books and magazines to start a library which tell you all about it.

3. You could also join—or start—a co-op and buy whole foods at a discount, again dividing the cost of purchase. I have found this plan very rewarding. You will have to ask others in your area where to find one, and if not available, start one!

4. You could also look for unused space for a cooperative garden to raise your own whole food which you *know* is not contaminated by poisonous sprays and chemicals. Be sure the space is not close to a highway where lead fumes can contaminate the plants.

I know a young woman who housecleans for others. She lives in a small trailer but has planted an organic garden on the property of a friend and there is enough food to exchange with the land owners instead of paying rent money for the garden space. The owners also provide the water.

HOW TO CURB YOUR FOOD BILLS

University experts insist that most people can cut their supermarket food bill fifteen percent by using the following tips:

• Never pay the full price for any food, they advise.

• Wait for sales and specials. Buy only when the price is right.

• Buy in quantity for future use. If an item is on sale, buy two, or if you can get someone to join you, buy 24.

• Compare sizes and contents on containers. Sometimes the larger size based on the unit cost, is cheaper in the long run.

• Store brands are often surprisingly cheaper than big name brands.

• Watch the newspaper for weekly specials and sales. If necessary, shop at competing stores. The money you will save will help pay for the extra gas you use.

• Plan meals around advertised specials. Don't buy beef if chicken is on sale. Be patient, the beef price drop will follow sooner or later. A turkey need not be for a Thanksgiving treat only. It supplies many leftover inexpensive meals including the final soup made from the carcass, embellished by bits and pieces of vegetables from your refrigerator: carrots, celery, parsley, etc.

• A pot roast can be stretched through several meals. Stews.

• Remember that organ meats are the most nutritious.

• Don't load up on carbohydrates or convenience foods like TV dinners. Make your own.

• Lastly, don't buy before a meal, when you are hungry. You will merely become an impulse buyer.

NOTES

1. Martin Zucker, "Bad Eating Makes Bad Marriages." *Let's LIVE* Magazine, March, 1979.

2. Marilyn Lambson, "To Life," *Let's LIVE* Magazine, March 1979.

3. Alexander G. Schauss, *Orthomolecular Treatment of Criminal Offenders*, published by Michael Lesser, M.D., President, Orthomolecular Medical Society, Berkeley, CA, 1978.

4. Martin Zucker, "Diet and Crime," *Let's LIVE* Magazine, May, 1979.

5. Dr. Leonard J. Hippchen, ed. *Ecologic-Biochemical Approaches to Treatment of Delinquents and Criminals.* New York: Van Nostrand, Reinhold, 1978.

6. Sandra Gibson, *Beyond the Body.* New York: Belmont Tower Books, 1979.

7. John Diamond, M.D., *BK: Behavorial Kinesiology,* New York: Harper and Row, 1979.

8. Linda Clark, *Stay Young Longer.* New York: Pyramid Publications, 1968.

CHAPTER TWELVE

Outwitting Addictions:
Alcohol, Sugar, Coffee, Tobacco

At the beginning of a recent food series in a magazine, now included in this book, the following letter arrived:

Dear Linda:

What is the nutritional answer for drug addiction? I am interested in the natural (herbal, naturopathic, nutritional, or scientific) way to stop taking drugs. This means cigarettes, alcohol, coffee, pot (marijuana), even refined (junk) foods; meats and dairy products (processed)—the whole gamut. There must be *some* health program available.

I am looking forward to an answer.

Thank you
(name deleted for privacy)

My answer:

"I believe I can help you outwit most addictions nutritionally except the proteins you mention. This is another story altogether, as you will soon discover."

How do such addictions begin? In the case of sugar, alcohol and coffee, your body usually craves or needs *something,* you are not quite sure what. So you begin to lean on something—anything—as a crutch to give you relief or a pickup. In general, sugar, alcohol and coffee belong to the same addiction family. All give you a temporary lift, but once used, they call for more, (to raise your blood sugar) and can become habit-forming. The more you have, the more you want. Fortunately, the reverse is also true: the less you have, the less you require. Better yet, when that missing factor or deficiency is supplied you may shed your dependence on such a crutch. Let's start with alcohol.

ALCOHOL

Not only do the causes of these addictions have much in common, but often there are similarities in their treatment. Willpower may help. But lack of willpower is usually *not* the root of the addiction. In fact, if the cause of the addiction is properly diagnosed and treated, willpower may not be needed at all, despite what others may think.

Not all people are addicts, as you know. Some can take a drink of alcohol, coffee, or a taste of sugar without craving more. These are the normal ones. For others, one taste is just a come-on, like eating peanuts; once you start you can't stop. Here among the addictive items is often a hidden or unrecognized deficiency. In the case of alcohol, sugar or coffee, your body may be trying to tell you it *needs* something. Meanwhile you are filling the need in the wrong way, thus perpetuating the addiction. You have heard of sugarholics and coffeeholics, as well as alcoholics. If you are one of these, just remember that willpower is *not* the only answer, if it is an answer at all, so stop feeling guilty. (Others are usually too quick to blame you in this respect.)

Here is what really happens: Because your body is crying for that something, alcohol, sugar or coffee makes you feel temporarily better; but you may fail to notice that the "good" reaction does not last. Before long you are feeling worse again. As you take more and more, you are trapped as if by quicksand. In order to extricate yourself permanently, you've got to find and supply the missing factor in order to get on top of the addiction. What is it? Here are some answers:

A MAJOR CAUSE OF ALCOHOLISM

Dr. Melvin Page, D.D.S., a specialist in endocrinology (gland therapy), classifies alcoholism as an illness. He considers it due to glandular insufficiency. He also believes that a well person cannot drink.

On the other hand, Roger J. Williams, Ph.D., an internationally known nutrition researcher and former director of the Clayton Bio-chemical Institute, University of Texas, has actually found the missing elements in alcoholics. His tests with rats revealed that the rats which were poorly nourished craved more alcohol than those which were well nourished. Furthermore, when certain nutritional elements were given to the alcohol-craving rats, they lost their craving! This observation has now been confirmed in hundreds of humans![1]

Since the rats do not know the meaning of "willpower," this should help an alcoholic overcome a feeling of guilt and attack the problem nutritionally. Dr. Williams gives examples:

Some wives who added these missing nutritional element into their husband's food or beverage so that the drinker was unaware of it were ecstatic to see the alcoholism disappear.

One case Dr. Williams cited was that of a graduate student in his own department. This man, due to his overwhelming craving for alcohol, was about to give up his graduate degree. But when he confided in Dr. Williams, who supplied the missing nutritional elements, the student's craving stopped and he earned his degree with no further trouble.

An entire chapter in my *Handbook of Natural Remedies for Common Ailments,*[2] is devoted to alcoholism. The exact nutrient products used by Dr. Williams, hopefully still available, follow:

Nutricol Forte—Vitamin Quota, 1125 Crenshaw Blvd., Los Angeles, CA 90019

G-154 Nutrins—General Nutrition Corp., 418 Weed Street, Pittsburgh, PA 15222

Glutamine—Erex Health Products, P.O. Box 178, Bernhart, MO 63012. L-Glutamine is also available in health stores.

Meanwhile, no doubt the psychiatrists and psychologists are upset because I have not given them due credit for locating the major cause or providing a cure of alcoholism. If the cause is emotional, psychiatry can, of course, be helpful. However, Dr. Williams found that in people, as well as in animals, alcoholics display a disturbed *physical* cellular metabolism which showed that some—perhaps most—alcoholics were suffering from a form of malnutrition. Alcoholism further complicates the problem since excessive drinking washes the B vitamins out of the body and B vitamins are needed to protect nerves. Alcoholics also soon begin to substitute drink for food, thereby increasing their malnutrition.

This information does not preclude other helps for alcoholism, such as Alcoholics Anonymous, Alanon, and psychiatry. As you know, alcoholism wears many different hats. Some alcoholics become very high and happy. Others become morose, depressed, vicious, sometimes violent, dangerous or even suicidal. Some will steal the family money to buy another drink. Still others will talk non-stop, or get sleepy, or perhaps be unable to sleep at all. Some become chronic complainers, shout and yell; others are impotent or sexually overstimulated, or sometimes become insanely jealous. Most alcoholics are generally irritable. No wonder a family member, for self-protection, tries to pack the alcoholic off to the nearest psychiatrist, just to get a little relief. If possible, try the dietary regimens first.

Why? Dr. Williams contends:

"I have seen too many serious alcoholics who had happy homes, were happy with their jobs, and appeared less in need of escape than most—yet were definitely alcoholics," meaning that alcoholism *can* be due to physical as well as emotional causes.

Alcoholics may be somewhat related to sugarholics who can't stop eating sugar, to coffeeholics who can't stop with one cup of coffee, or smokers who find that one cigarette leads to another. There may well be a physiological cause for all. For example, Dr. Williams learned that the hypothalamus, a portion of the brain related to appetite control has been mildly poisoned by alcohol. You will soon learn that sugarholism and or coffeeholism can be caused by, or be the outgrowth of, another malfunctioning gland, the pancreas, and what to do about it. Here is Dr. William's general program for alcoholics and it may help the sugarholics and coffeeholics, too:

1. Plenty of good protein—dairy products,including eggs, and fish, poultry, meat or other rich sources of protein.

2. Vegetables—both green and yellow; raw and cooked.

3. Fat in some form—natural oils, butter, nuts, grains, etc.

4. Avoidance of processed or junk foods which are usually deficient or completely lacking in vitamins, minerals and other nutrients. White sugar is a striking example.

5. Plenty of rest.

6. Regular indoor and outdoor exercise to help circulation to, and regeneration of, the hypothalamus.

Dr. Williams also believes in ALL vitamins/minerals, not a separate one here and there. He likens them all to links of a chain, although it is well-known that the B vitamins are particularly important in alcoholism.

Dr. Williams has also found that a nonessential amino acid *glutamine* (a protein) has provided quick results for many alcoholics. He tells of one long standing case of alcoholism in which, on a doctor's prescription, the glutamine was added to the victim's drinking water without his knowledge. The person stopped drinking promptly without any side effects. (Glutamine is not the same as glutamic acid.)[2]

Several years ago, a psychiatrist, Jack Cooper, M.D., developed a different nutritional program for chronic alcoholics in a New York state penitentiary. The tests continued for ten years, during which time the number of cases of D.T.s (delerium tremens) and alcoholic convulsions ceased dramatically. Dr. Cooper first began with a high protein drink, and of course, being a psychiatrist, he applied psychiatric help to the patients, too. But he was not completely satisfied with results. Finally he evolved a nutritional formula which at that time, in his search for help for alcholics, proved to be the best to date.

The Formula ("Cooper Cocktail"):

A combination of magnesium, vitamin B_6, brewer's yeast, niacin and vitamin C, plus calcium. Although some of the forms of these ingredients he used were, at the time, uncommon, he was on the right track and ahead of his time. Health stores now stock these ingredients in more acceptable forms and other researchers are learning that they are helpful for various types of addiction, including alcoholism.

Still later, Dr. Cooper, not yet completely satisfied with the results of his Cooper Cocktail, eventually turned to homeopathy with better results.[3]

Some investigators blame heredity for alcoholism. This may be true, but poor nutrition and its results may also be inherited. One example: it is now well-known that some alcoholic mothers are giving birth to babies with alcohol on their breath, and therefore, are already on the alcoholic path. In fact, whatever the mother's addiction, it is usually passed on to the child. A researcher of biological science at Carnegie-Mellon University reports genetic as well as permanent brain damage due to alcoholism.

Nutrition is a simple and painless method of reversing alcoholism, and since it may well supply the "missing factor" causing the problem, is certainly worth a try. Those who have witnessed the good results give testimony to its good effects.

THE COFFEE-SUGAR CONNECTION

Sugar tastes good to many people. Others find it sickening. Children usually love sugar—and parents, knowing this, have long used it as a reward. In England, school teachers have even rewarded or quieted students by passing around a box of "sweets." Tea time in England or its colonies is usually based on sweets: scones with jams, cakes, tarts and the like. As a result, the general condition of most Britishers' teeth is considered disastrous. And now Dr. John Yudkin of England has warned that sugar is also a possible cause of heart attacks.

In the United States, in addition to cavities, such physiological disorders as diabetes and hypolgycemia appear to be commonplace penalties for eating an oversweet diet. Commercial companies, anxious to make money, know that adults as well as children usually love sweets too, so they overload many foods with it. Reading your labels is necessary to avoid extra sugar in such foods as chewing gum, soft drinks, jams, jellies, fruit juices, canned fruits, etc., as well as the usual desserts. A teaspoon of sugar here and there can soon add up to many cupfuls although you may believe you do not eat much sugar at all. It even lurks in some peanut butter, catsup, bottled salad dressings, crackers, artificial cream whips and non-dairy creamers, as well as in bouillon cubes, gelatins, so-called "100% natural" cereals, candy bars, cakes, cookies, frozen fruit-flavor bars, and on and on.

And be especially careful of those labels which shout, "Sugarless!" The products may not be made with sugar, but they may contain other sweeteners. Xylitol, sorbitol and mannitol are among the substitutes often used. They are known as sugar alcohols, and contain as many calories as sucrose (regular sugar). Fructose, previously discussed, is another type of sugar.

Corn syrup too, (also known as glucose and dextrose), though innocent sounding, has been found in a study to cause a serious type of diabetes. Corn syrup is less sweet so more is added to a food without its being detected. It is also absorbed more rapidly than other sugars. Due to the fact it is possible to consume it in larger amounts unknowingly, corn syrup was at one time banned in Canada for use in sweet drinks. [4] It is *not* banned in the U.S. and I personally refuse to buy a product which contains it. Read labels for protection.

WHAT STARTED YOUR SUGAR ADDICTION?

Parents, grandparents and well-meaning friends often indulge children with sweets for various reasons. In sports, many coaches formerly gave their athletes sugar or candy bars to increase their energy. Even doctors and dentists have been guilty of giving children lollipops as a "reward." My own children, denied commercial sugars at home, discovered candy Easter eggs at a party.

Why is sugar so treacherous? Because it raises the blood sugar too quickly, makes you feel good at first until your blood sugar nose-dives soon afterwards, whereupon you feel far worse than before. The victim then grabs more sugar to restore the "good feeling" or energy lift and the whole thing becomes a yo-yo.

But, more importantly, sugar stimulates the pancreas to produce insulin, and the number one ailment in America today is called hyperinsulinism, low blood sugar, or hypoglycemia. Continuous reports state that nearly every one is afflicted with it to some degree. It can cause headaches, weakness, fatigue, shakiness, particularly irritability, mental confusion and even blackouts, as well. The pancreas, which becomes trigger-happy due to the constant exposure to sugar, becomes so skittish it loses its balance and researchers state that it can eventually lead the victim of hypoglycemia down the road to a full-fledged case of diabetes. Protein can raise the blood sugar safely, more slowly. The effects lasts longer.

Hypoglycemia has definitely been controlled by a high protein, no sugar diet, with *NO coffee.* (Very weak tea is allowed.) Why is coffee a no-no in hypoglycemia? When you drink a cup of coffee, the pancreas thinks, "Here comes a meal and I am supposed to manufacture a load of insulin to handle it." But there is no meal forthcoming to use that insulin; the coffee is a false alert. If this continues, the overstimulated pancreas becomes tired, lazy, weaker, and eventually may refuse to work at all. So the stage for diabetes has been set. Dr. Bruce Pacetti, a nutritionist, considers sugar a form of slow suicide. And hear this: *any sweet,* as well as coffee, *can trick the pancreas into an overproduction of insulin.* Even though the high-protein hypoglycemic diet can help get your pancreas back in working order by providing a vacation from all the stimulating sugar and/or coffee, the pancreas apparently never forgets. One woman remained on a hypoglycemic, no sugar, no coffee, high-protein diet for three years and then decided she was cured. She drank one cup of coffee and the disturbance returned in a flash!

WHAT ABOUT SUGAR SUBSTITUTES?

Sugar substitutes merely keep your sugar craving alive and continue to fool the pancreas. Most people can substitute safely a *little* fresh raw fruit when a sugar craving hits them. Meanwhile they can begin cutting down the sugar content of their foods gradually and eventually wean themselves of the craving.

If you feel you *must* have teaspoon after teaspoon of sugar in your tea, begin by cutting out one teaspoon at a time. Women can begin to lower sugar in recipes, and serve fresh fruits as substitutes for pies, cakes and other desserts. Before long, you will be surprised how sickening oversweet foods can taste. One family I know began by having dessert on Saturday nights only, rather than daily at dinner time, and finally dropped that weekly "treat" too, without any family member complaining.

HOW TO SIDESTEP COFFEE

After understanding the effect of coffee on the pancreas (caffeine is considered the culprit) you no doubt may decide to replace coffee with substitutes, including tea, decaffeinated coffee and herb teas. Wait, until you read the whole story here! Tea also contains caffeine, although weak tea is allowed on the hypoglycemic diet.

Some people who are getting off large amounts of coffee may substitute dozens of cups of herb tea daily. Herbs, in large amounts may also be a hazard to some people. Herbs were our earliest medicines, and though considered safer today than drugs, still may actively or gradually disagree with some people. They are most beneficial when used with moderation.[5] I have never known a well-trained herbalist to dispute this advice. Chosen with care for *you,* a few daily cups of herb tea are probably OK.

Decaffeinated coffee has long been in use for those who recognized a possible threat from regular coffee, but many people have complained that for them the side effects of decaffeinated coffee were worse than those of regular coffee. The symptoms apparently include weakness, shakiness, as well as a general feeling of malaise. This may be explained by the chemical solvent (methylenechloride) used by manufacturers to remove the caffeine, leaving some of the residue in the decaffeinated product.

Good news has arrived! There is a new Swiss method of removing caffeine *without* chemical solvents.

The new decaffeinating process consists of using real coffee beans from which the caffeine is removed by a fresh water bath before drying, roasting and grinding the beans. For a source of supply, write: Customer Relations Department, The White Coffee Corporation, Box 1092/11-50, 44th Road, Long Island City, New York 11101.

There is also the cold water extraction type of coffee essence which some people can use. A special portable appliance is available at various hardware, kitchen supply, and department stores. You allow the cold water to cover the ground coffee and steep all night, removing the grains the following morning and refrigerating the essence which is added as needed, a tablespoon to a cup of boiling water. Fats and toxins of the coffee are said to be eliminated by this method. Try it. If you become shaky a short time later, even this form of coffee is not for you. Your pancreas has objected (the cause of the shakiness). Each person, being different, must find his or her own beverage as well as the amount which can be tolerated.

HOW TO STOP DRINKING COFFEE

Most people who have already given up coffee warn others not to give it up suddenly. The body does not like sudden changes, and excruciating headaches have resulted from a sudden cessation of coffee. Begin by cutting out one cup at a time. Then drink only a half cup, then a third, a fourth, until you can give it up entirely.

One hazard when you are trying to stop is eating at a restaurant. Some restaurants, in spite of the rising cost of coffee, still fill up your cup when you aren't looking. The way out of this dilemma is to turn your cup upside down when you are ready to call a halt, and the waiter will get the message.

In any case, *coffee should never be taken alone.* It provides too much stress for the pancreas. The same is true if taken with a sweet "Danish" for breakfast. Protein is better to take with coffee than taking it with a sweet or alone. Protein acts as a buffer. Nuts, seeds, cubes of cheese are some protein possibilities.

At coffee-break time in the office bring your own can of vacuum packed sunflower seeds (which are delicious as well as nutritious—the vacuum pack avoids rancidity). Or bring your own nuts, cheese, even popcorn, and don't complain if the other workers gobble them up. Ask them to contribute similar goodies next time. This is a sure way, incidentally, to prevent that four o'clock slump, often the result of a steady parade throughout the day to the office coffee machine.

Believe it or not, once you have kicked the coffee habit, you not only feel great (ask anyone who has done it and is no longer a slave to the brew). You even reach the stage that though it gives off a captivating fragrance while brewing, when you actually taste it, it tastes awful! Hard to believe, but true.

SMOKING

I wish I could be as encouraging about smoking as about alcohol withdrawal. Although there are definite ways out, the victim must *want* to quit! No one can make another do it. Hints, nagging and ultimatums merely make smokers more stubborn. They insist that they can do whatever they want to do. Sure they can, but they might stop to think of others. They may be seriously endangering the health of those around them, even killing them, but their determination to smoke blindly keeps them from thinking of anyone else but themselves. The effects of smoking have been found to create serious problems for others as well as the smoker.

Also, *smoking can cause:*

1. Heart attacks
2. Radioactivity and other contaminations from many pollutants
3. Carbon monoxide poisoning
4. Nicotine poisoning (also used as a poison in insectides)
5. Emphysema, bronchitis and cancer (and can irritate asthma)
6. A decline in vision within twenty minutes after smoking a cigarette
7. Lack of oxygen to various body parts, including lungs and the brain
8. Ulcers
9. Slowed reflexes
10. Wrinkles and appearance of aging skin

11. Allergies
12. Baldness

Smokers forget that they affect others by exposing them to the whole list of ailments above. Heart attacks in children have been reported due to their parents' smoking.

Dr. Alfred Munzer, President of the District of Columbia Lung Association, as well as serving as lung specialist for the Washington, D.C. Adventist hospital, states that the effect of parental smoking on children is equivalent to a child smoking from three to five cigarettes a day. (Max Huberman, *Health Food Retailing,* October 1979)

In addition, a medical study conducted by the School of Medicine University of California, San Diego, revealed that a pregnant woman who smokes can stunt her baby's growth, cause hyperactivity, and seriously impair the child's learning ability. (*United Press.* October 9, 1979).

Wrinkles in men or women do not show up immediately, but later in life their skin resembles a washboard. I have seen it happen, particularly in women.

I, personally, am allergic to tobacco smoke and can suffer from nicotine poisoning after exposure to smoking by others, whether in a car, plane, a private home, including my own, a restaurant, or a supermarket. Deliver me from a cigar! I can smell a cigar from one end of a huge supermarket to the other. And I have seen women who were smoking near a shelf or counter in a supermarket where I was shopping notice me flinch and defiantly blow smoke into my face. I assure you a tobacco allergy is rough, and is not due to imagination.

Meanwhile I feel deeply for others subjected to the same thoughtless treatment by their companions. One woman wrote me not once, but several times, saying piteously, "I would give *anything* if there were an herb or *something* which would help my husband lose his taste for tobacco." I know of no herb, if there is one, but you can look at other withdrawal methods I will list later.

One couple suddenly noticed an unexplained bronchitis in both of them. It turned out to be caused by the man who smoked heavily (the woman did not). But did he stop? No! I always warn people not to nag their husbands, wives or companions. It will only make them worse.

In a professional club, I will never forget the case of one couple.

The man smoked like a chimney. Even his wife admitted that their carpets, drapery and furniture at home were supersaturated with tobacco smoke. Apparently his wife (a non-smoker) was not allergic to it. Her husband proudly told all his friends, "My wife *never* criticizes my smoking; she actually encourages me to continue." Mrs. Goody-Two-Shoes evidently considered it very masculine for her husband to smoke and every man in the club went home and held that wife up as a shining example of a tolerant attitude to her husband's smoking—that is, until he suddenly died of a massive heart attack.

Due to public pressure there are attempts to ban smoking in some restaurants, food stores and planes, or at least to set up safety islands for those who do not smoke and suffer from the smoke from those who so.

Don Matchan, author of the book, *We Do Mind If You Smoke,* tells of one wife who became extremely ill when going into smoky places. She eventually was forced to turn down invitations to homes where smoking was allowed, and to make advance reservations in restaurants with smokefree areas when she and her husband went out to dine. At first this oversensitivity irritated her husband until he witnessed how ill the smoke from others made her. Then he became angry at their thoughtlessness and took up the cudgel for his wife.[6]

In my own home I have met with full cooperation from friends and business associates who visit me. I tell them when they arrive that I am allergic to tobacco smoke and ask them to smoke outdoors. They do.

Don Matchan suggests that the next time you are exposed to a human smokestack or one who asks if you mind if they smoke, tell the truth, or whip out a 3"x5" card prepared in advance, which reads: "Pardon me, but would you mind blowing your hydroquinone, methacrolein, methyl alcohol, methylamine, nickel compounds, pyridine, carbon monoxide, carbon dioxide, crotonitrile, dimethylamine, endrin, ethylamine, furfural, cadmium, methyl nitrate, ammonia, formaldehyde, hydrogen sulfide, benzo (a) pyrene, nicotine, DDT, ethane, acetylene, methanol, nitrogen dioxide, acetone, methyl chloride, phenol, cresol, methane, isoprene, propane, acrolein, acetaldyde, ethylene, methyl ethyl ketone, tar, hydrogen cyanide, hydrocyanic acid, nitric, acetonitrile, bezene, 2,3,butdione, and butylamine in the other direction?''

For those who wonder why our forefathers and the American Indians were healthy in spite of heavy smoking, here is your answer. These contaminants were not known in earlier days, nor were they present in the air, soil or water as tobacco growing mediums, which tobacco now absorbs. ''Civilization'' has caught up with us!

HOW SMOKING ADDICTIONS START

How and why do smoking addictions start? You know the answer as well as I do: Social Pressures; it is ''the thing to do.'' Teenagers do it to appear more adult to their friends. Adults do it because VIPs do it. (I have news for you. Many VIPs are trying desperately to stop!) Years ago the tobacco companies wished to sell more tobacco. So they enlisted women smokers by placing pictures of beautiful women smoking on large billboards across the highways of America. That did it! One by one, women became hooked. Many are still hooked, and probably don't know why. Once you start, it becomes a habit and you wish to heaven you had never started.

Smoking also has a psychological factor. It becomes something you can do with your hands and mouth to hide your tensions and insecurity. To me a smoker who grabs a cigarette as a crutch, in reality hoists a sign which reads: ''I AM INSECURE. SMOKING HELPS ME APPEAR MORE NORMAL (or attractive, or important).''

The cancer label of the surgeon general at first worried the tobacco companies. But the public apparently ignores it now and the tobacco companies have breathed a sigh of relief. They are still somewhat nervous, however, since many smokers are trying to stop. They are pulling out every possible advertising stop to halt such a blow to their prestige and pockets.

KICKING THE HABIT

In Don Matchan's book, *We Do Mind If You Smoke,* his chapter on kicking the habit contains helpful suggestions for quitting. There is insufficient space here to enumerate them, but he does say that quitting cold turkey may be the easiest. Others agree. The gradual method may have fewer side effects, but it prolongs the agony and makes that remaining cigarette more enjoyable. He suggests these tips to help: when the craving becomes unbearable, take a drink of water, or look at your watch, wait one minute before yielding to the next cigarette. Exercise helps reduce tension, too. He also lists a five-day withdrawal plan. I have included a breathing method, outlined step by step, in my book, *Rejuvenation.* Those who have tried it claim that it is successful.

A new method, reported by the *National Enquirer,* June 1979, claims that the University of Nebraska's College of Medicine found that 82.4 percent of whose who added ordinary baking soda tablets to their diet were able to kick the smoking habit in four weeks. I do not know whether this works or not. Raw vegetables for which I opt were also reported as achieving similar results.

Many reformed smokers say they found it easier to quit if there were no cigarettes kept on the premises to tempt them.

If you simply must have help, the Schick Centers, one of the most widely advertised professional methods, guarantee to stop your smoking or your money is refunded. They claim they have helped over fifty thousand people become nonsmokers. Since the method is recommended by a doctor, your doctor's office might be able to give you the location of the Center in your area. Or look in the yellow pages of your phone book.

The fact that smokers who do quit, often gain weight is explained by a temporary upset in metabolism, which eventually adjusts to normal, as does the weight. But be careful of food substitutes you choose to pamper yourself in the meantime. One nutritionist, who should have known better, told me she indulged in candy and sweets while quitting smoking and developed a crop of cavities. Watch out also for overconsumption of stimulating drinks—alcohol, coffee and tea. Raw foods, small meals eaten often, and a hypoglycemia high-protein diet have helped many. Give your body all the nutrients it needs, especially calcium and B vitamins to calm your nervous system. Protein should provide needed energy to substitute for the lift you have been getting from your smoke. Zinc is also said to help.

Don Matchan reports good results through meditation and prayer. Whatever helps you make the grade, the reward for purging yourself of the smoking urge is *great,* according to those who have kicked the habit.

NOTES

1. Roger J. Williams, Ph.D., *Alcoholism: The Nutritional Approach.* Austin, TX: University of Texas Press. 1959. For some reason this little book has been either ignored or overlooked. If your bookstore cannot find it write directly to the publisher for information at Box 7819, University Station, Austin, TX 78712.

2. Linda Clark, *Handbook of Natural Remedies for Common Ailments.* New York: Pocket Books, 1978. Available in paperback and hard cover through health and book stores.

3. Dr. Callavardin, Lyons, France, *How to Cure Alcoholim—The Non-Toxic Homeopathic Way.* Translated from the French. Available from East-West Arts, Ltd., P.O. Box 85, Katonah, NY 10536.

4. Frances Lukens, M.D., and Curtis Dohan, M.D.U., of Pennsylvania. *Endocrinology,* Vol. 42, 1948, p. 244. See also, Linda Clark, *Stay Young Longer,* Chapter Seven: Is Sugar Harmful?

5. Linda Clark, *How To Improve Your Health: The Wholistic Approach to Health.* New Canaan, CT: Keats Publishing, Inc., 1979. See chapter on herbs and herb teas.

6. Don C. Matchan, *We Mind If You Smoke.* New York: Pyramid Publications, 1977. Don Matchan is editor of the National Health Federation Bulletin, is a nutritional student and a long-time respected newspaper writer. This book is built on solid, documented facts, not mere fancy.

CHAPTER THIRTEEN

Drug Addiction—Ways Out

The reader who wrote to me recently for help in getting off drugs (pot) is apparently a rare exception. In my search for answers to help this reader and others outwit marijuana and other drug addictions, I learned that most addicts—be it pot, heroin, "speed" (amphetamines), LSD or "uppers"—do not want to get off drugs! There is little use, then, in trying to convert them until they are ready. I hope the following information will speed their desire to withdraw.

One pot (marijuana) addict pulled himself out after being motivated by the shock of witnessing the death of his cousin, a girl who had not made the withdrawal and eventually committed suicide. The addict, on seeing her dead in her coffin, asked, "Do I want to continue to go my way or hers?" He decided to kick the habit, used the nutritional method for withdrawal, and today has a successful and exciting career. He looks and feels great.

Drug addicts admit they became hooked because they wanted status or acceptance from others who indulged. Drug peddlers also make many conquests which liberally increases their income.

Those who start smoking marijuana apparently believe at first that it makes life easier and more amusing. Later they admit that the amusing effects eventually wear off and life's problems seem to get worse instead of better. As they begin to feel worse they frantically use more and more pot until they usually can no longer sleep or function efficiently. Nevertheless, they continue to lean on pot for false energy. Among other problems is the historical fact that, like alcoholics, they become notoriously unsafe drivers, a potential hazard to everyone on the highway. Therapists who have worked with addicts in drug rehabilitation centers state that marijuana can cause a complete personality change: users often become inveterate liars, cheats, thieves—completely unstable individuals—often going through one relationship after another, a shifting job picture, and suffering from gradually increasing illness and depression.

One man who did recover said he tried to give up his addiction and for three days felt absolutely dead. This convinced him something was wrong with traditional withdrawal systems. He finally got on the nutritional cure program, and is now on his way to becoming a Ph.D. and a veterinarian, goals to which he had long aspired. I will later give you the details of his nutritional withdrawal diet which he willingly shares with audiences.

Another addict, a former schizophrenic and victim of general addictions to sugar and alcohol as well as to drugs, is an orthomolecular psychiatrist. (Orthomolecular refers to the use of varying dosages, sometimes massive, of certain vitamins and minerals, plus a good nutritional diet, all under medical supervision.)

He has told how even a small glass of wine, beer or hard liquor set up in him a craving for more. Since he is a doctor and had access to free drug samples, he admits he became hooked on dexedrine, increasing his daily intake until he was downing 104 dexedrine tablets *alone* on the 104th day. By this time he was gobbling a *total* of 450 tablets of various drugs daily. Eventually he became a nervous wreck, lost his medical license and, though at one time a millionaire, ended up, he says, in the Salvation Army.

Through nutrition and orthomolecular treatment he finally succeeded in pulling himself out, retrieved his medical license, and as the reinstated medical director of a state medical hospital in California, began helping other addicts. His statistics are shocking. He states there are hundreds of doctors, nurses and hospital workers who are drug addicts—or were, only to become suicides, with the cause of death listed (especially in the case of doctors) as ''heart attack'' (a cover-up on death certificates). He also reports the good news that in this country as of 1975, there were already 48,000 recovered alcoholics and 18,000 recovered drug addicts.

To date there are few nutrition-oriented rehabilitation centers for drug addiction withdrawal treatments. Some psychiatrists, who have been rehabilitated by this nutritional method, are convinced it's not only the coming thing, but a sure thing in drug addiction rehabilitation. It certainly is far easier than other, more rugged, measures.

Recovered addicts warn that the fact "pot" is being legalized in some areas—and even recommended for various diseases—should not be relied upon as an alibi for indiscriminate use, which could end in addiction. In fact, researchers, as well as recovered addicts, report that marijuana is often the first step to later and more serious hard drug addiction, including heroin, often leading to fatal consequences such as that described at the end of this chapter, a gripping, never-to-be-forgotten story according to those who have heard it.

PROGRAMS FOR OUTWITTING ADDICTION

Even though there seems to be a lack of nutritional rehabilitation centers for drug addiction (a situation which should be remedied immediately), there are nutritional researchers and doctors who have already used this method successfully for their patients.

Carlton Fredericks, Ph.D., nutrition researcher and teacher, says in his book, *The Nutrition Handbook: Your Key to Good Health,* "In both drug addiction and alcoholism there is a need for good nutrition. Since both groups suffer from the impact of their self-chosen, poor diet, they can be helped physically and mentally by a high-protein diet of hypoglycemia type, with multiple vitamins, multiple minerals and the B vitamins, both in concentrated supplemental form, plus the special purpose foods—such as desiccated liver, brewer's yeast and the like."

Drs. E. Cheraskin and W. M. Ringsdorf, Jr., with Arlene Brecher in their book *Psycho-Dietetics,* provide some invaluable information for addictions of many kinds—coffee, sugar, alcohol, and hard drugs as well as marijuana. These authors show why diet probably became so poor in the first place.

They also show how many doctor-given drugs can produce a deficiency of nutrients. For example, drug sedatives can cause a deficiency of multiple vitamins, especially vitamin D (needed for calcium absorption, a natural nerve sedative).

There are other hazards, especially with oral contraceptives, which, according to these authors, creates a body loss of at least "four essential brain-cell nutrients: vitamin B_1, folic acid, vitamin B_{12} and vitamin C." These losses of nutrients can result in insomnia, fatigue, nervousness and depression, lethargy, and other symptoms. Such doctor-administered drugs have been found to lead to dependence on other drugs, according to the *Psycho-Dietetics* book.

The authors conclude, "Most people believe the nation's real drug problem to be our young people's . . . abuse . . . of the mind-expanding drugs. Less well-known are the promising results achieved in rehabilitating young drug addicts by nutritional therapy . . . and their return to normal living."

The book outlines the authors' *Optimal Diet* which includes high-protein foods containing all amino acids in balance: meat, fish, fowl, eggs, cheese, certified raw or cultured milk, plus vitamins and minerals, particularly niacin (a B vitamin) and massive doses of C under medical supervision, both vitamins capable of dramatic results. This book lists much more excellent, practical help for overcoming addictions, including the warning to eat sparingly of commercially tampered-with foods. Junk foods, of course, are *out*. (If you don't buy them, you won't be tempted to eat them.)

Foods to avoid are completely refined white sugar and white flour, additives and preservatives, such as nitrates and nitrites. Of all the foods to be avoided, the most harmful, according to these authors, is white sugar.

Dr. Alfred Libby, following the lead of Dr. Irwin Stone, from whom Dr. Linus Pauling discovered the importance of vitamin C, concentrates on huge doses of vitamin C for addicts (used under medical supervision) because the results are both quick and without side or withdrawal effects. The form of vitamin C used by these doctors with great success for narcotic addicts is sodium ascorbate, which apparently detoxifies the body even after years of stress resulting from addiction.

Dr. Libby's detoxification-nutritional treatment of drug addiction does not stop with vitamin C. He recommends whole, natural foods, high-protein meals, and an abundance of vitamin and mineral supplements. He forbids junk foods, such as white bread, desserts, sodas, and donuts, while encouraging fresh vegetables, natural raw juices, and meat. The reason for meat is that he discovered his addicted patients lacked ten important amino acids in their urine, suggestive of a disease known as *kwashiorkor,* caused by nutritional deficiencies, especially of protein. He also points out that dosages of any supplements can vary from addict to addict which is a concept of Dr. Roger Williams and based on individual differences. You can read more on Dr. Libby's successful work in the reversal of drug addiction in *Let's LIVE,* October 1978).

The man who is now studying to become a veterinarian mentioned earlier, recovered from his addiction by taking, under medical supervision, large doses of niacin daily for three years. He learned that vitamins and minerals taken instead of drugs, satisfied his release from the unpleasant symptoms of drugs. He says that a good nutritional diet plus vitamins B_6 and B_{12} and potassium, plus meditation and yoga (which help his anxiety problems) keep him feeling fit and well. He follows the suggestion of Alanon (Alcoholics Anonymous) of taking one day at a time.

The psychiatrist states that orthomolecular or megavitamins returned him to his feeling of normalcy *in three days.* In the case of niacin, the "flushing" reaction for which it is known (which is actually only a histamine-release process) soon disappears on continued use. He warns against allergies to certain seafoods such as shrimp and lobster, which in some addicts can cause violent reactions. He also warns against the use of sugar and sleeping pills, as well as tranquilizers such as valium which, in itself, can cause a drug addiction. For himself, he still uses, along with other nutrients, niacin, B_6 and B_{12} as well as vitamin E.

A MORE RECENT APPROACH

In my opinion, the most exciting help of all is being provided by Alexander G. Schauss, who treats both criminal offenders and drug addicts with nutrition. If this connection startles you, don't forget that much crime and delinquency has followed a poor diet, and that criminal offense might be perhaps just a hop-skip-and-a-jump away from drug addiction.

Delinquencies, at least, and even murders and other crimes, have been traced to both poor diet and/or drug addiction. Mental aberrations can occur, although the exact cause may be hard to pinpoint at the time. Those of the younger generation who have seen such movies as "Rosemary's Baby," "The Exorcist," "The Omen," and others do not argue the presence of the message to be found there. Remember the young man who climbed the tower at the University of Texas and took potshots at innocent passing students, killing an incredible number? Prior to this deranged behavior, which resulted in his death he had confided to doctors, "I hear voices that tell me to do things."

Such crimes are increasing rather than decreasing. Yet Barbara Reed, of Ohio, found a common denominator of poor diet—mainly hypoglycemia—underlying the causes of misdemeanors. When treated by nutrition, they did not recur.

Alexander Schauss, a thirty-year-old genius, is a comparative newcomer to this field, having entered it recently after a brilliant career as a training officer with the Washington State Corrections Training program. At 21 he became the youngest probation-parole officer in New Mexico's history.

Alex Schauss noticed while dealing with criminal offenders or drug addicts that those who were able to kick their fast foods and junk foods diet were also able to kick their drug addictions or criminal tendencies. His excellent program for either drug addiction or criminal offense is based on a "sound mind in a sound body." He has shown by actual tests that those who ate fresh, unprocessed foods, used no tea, coffee, or refined sugar, and snacked often on whole nutritional foods, were rehabilitated. He also recommends daily exercise, summer and winter, to tone up the body, improve circulation and maintain optimum all around fitness.

He believes that lack of natural light, as explained by Dr. John Ott, is another factor in mind and body aberrations. He encourages hair testing for locating heavy metal poisoning and mineral deficiencies which might be undermining health. His system works! He is now training over seven hundred professionals, including doctors, in using this program. His booklet, *Orthomolecular Treatment of Criminal Offenders,* describes his program, diet, and many case histories of success in criminal delinquency offering as well a number of proven suggestions for drug addiction withdrawal. He feels that anyone who wishes to pull himself out of an addiction *can do it*.

This booklet is now being expanded into a book *Diet and Delinquency* by Alexander G. Schauss, available from the Institute of Bio-Social Research, City College, Graduate School, Lyon Building, Seattle, Washington 98401. You may write this address for information about these publications, or for the name of the nearest center where addicts can get such help. Alex Schauss, in an article "Marijuana, Little Friend, Big Foe," published in *Let's Live,* August, 1979, by Harvey M. Ross, M.D., points out that the marijuana industry is said to gross from 20 to 48 billion dollars annually, and that marijuana is not the innocent substance it is claimed to be.

In fact, according to Dr. Ross, "Pot is beginning to rival the processed food industry as the number one health hazard."

Now to the reader who asked how to outwit "addictions to meat" you can see why I do not condemn these proteins, nor are they addictions. This question may well express a craving—or need for such foods. They have been used liberally in all successful drug withdrawals.

Finally, here is the story about the testimonial by a drug addict who taped his story, which was later made public on a chilling nationwide newscast. Craig (his last name no longer matters) was a university student and only seventeen when it happened. His last will and testament was a tape recording in which he told in detail the physical torment and mental anguish of his journey through drugs.

In tones of remorse and futility he warned other youngsters of the dangers of drugs, and bid farewell to his parents, and his friends. Then young Craig, once a university honor student, put to rest his torture. He drove into the Wyoming countyryside and "shot himself between the eyes." Reported months later in *Time* magazine (Nov. 22, 1970).

He had not had the benefit of nutrition to facilitate his withdrawal. Had he realized—and tried—it, there might have been another way out. One drug addict, now recovered, who tells me he personally knows hundreds of addicts. He says of the many successful recoveries from drug addiction he has never known any to succeed without spiritual help, including prayer and meditation.

NOTES

1. Carlton Fredericks, Ph.D., *Dr. Carlton Fredericks' New and Complete Nutrition Handbook: Your Key to Good Health.* Chatsworth, CA: Major Books, 1978.

2. E. Cheraskin and W. M. Ringsdorf, Jr. with Arlene Brecher, *Psycho-Dietetics.* New York: Bantam, 1976.

3. Alfred Libby, *Let's LIVE* Magazine, October, 1978.

4. Alexander G. Schauss, *Orthomolecular Treatment of Criminal Offenders.* published by Michael Lesser, M.D., President, Orthomolecular Medical Society, Berkeley, CA, 1978.

5. Alexander G. Schauss, *Diet and Delinquency,* available from the Institute of Bio-Social Research, City College, Graduate School, Lyon Building, Seattle, WA 98401.

CHAPTER FOURTEEN

A Health Secret

I will now share with you a most remarkable diet, based somewhat in general, on the primitive diets. It has helped many to normalize health and weight, especially overweight, and without hunger. But it does much more. It has also helped to reverse or prevent many ailments which may have long plagued you. They range from heart disease, diabetes, hardening of the arteries, high blood pressure, to gall stones, some urinary problems, allergies, and many more, as well as to achieve a "top of the world feeling" you may have forgotten you ever felt. Hypoglycemia just seems to disappear on this diet.

I, personally, am not making claims for this diet, merely reporting the findings of doctors (M.D.'s, not even natural therapists whom the orthodox organizations so often consider "unacceptable.") I have discovered that there have been between 69 to 79 or more medical physicians who swear to the success of this diet after trying it on various ailments in their patients.

It may come as no surprise that this diet is controversial, often because it is against the interests of some commercial groups, even uninformed doctors who have not learned, studied or used it, thus throw verbal stones at it. You may see many diatribes against it in newspapers, magazine articles and books. In fact, books which have been previously written about it by orthodox doctors in otherwise good standing, are now out of print, possibly a deliberately planned action? One explanation has been submitted by the late Blake F. Donaldson, M.D., who used the diet successfully in his own practice. He wrote in a book about the diet,[1] that what the nation is eating and buying is of great concern to commercial interests. He says, "A little woman pushing a cart through the country's shopping centers is the clue. What she buys or does not buy can make manufacturers tremble and governments totter.'' Yet, I repeat, that this diet was based in general upon one or more of the primitive tribes studied by Dr. Price, and has stood the test of time.

I must reiterate the statement made many times earlier, that due to individual difference, not everyone may be helped by this diet. However, the fact remains that hundreds of thousands of unsolicited testimonials have reached doctors who have used or written about it, and all were enthusiatic about the diet's success. So don't let criticisms and barbs influence you adversely. Try it fairly before you judge!

I first learned about this diet many years ago from Stefansson, the internationally famous anthropologist of Harvard University. Stef, as he was called, spent many years living and eating with the Eskimos in their native Arctic habitats. He wrote numerous books about what he learned and experienced there. He was delighted with the improvement in his own health on the Eskimo diet, as well as observing the tribe's good health as a whole, and returned enthusiastically to the United States with the information he had learned. Although he has told his story in his books, I was privileged to know him well up to the day before he died, at which time he was still upright, dying at a ripe old age with his boots on, of a quick and painless death. That last day with him before I left him in the East to fly West, he was showing me the manuscript of his final book, *Discovery*. Though you can find verification in his books of his diet findings, I believe you might find it more interesting to hear his story as he related it to me.

The diet on which the Eskimos lived was, believe it or not, a high fat, high protein diet, with little or no carbohydrates. He told me that the Eskimos at that time ate six parts of fat to one of protein, so he preferred to call it a high fat diet. The protein came mainly from fish, some caribou and any other animals they could find, whereas the fat came from seal blubber and oil. This form of fat was considered not only a delicacy but a must for health. You will recall the story I have already relayed from him how he and a companion, trekking across the tundra, had acquired excruciating headaches, until they met another traveller who discovered the two men had no fat to eat with their protein. On sharing some seal oil with them Stef said the headaches vanished almost immediately and never returned *as long as they continued to eat fat.*

On his return home, he continued to search for adequate fat, which I thought at the time was a bit "far out" but I later learned differently when I finally tried the diet myself.

Carbohydrates did not appear prominently in the Eskimo diet. In the summer, a few berries supplied vitamin C, but the main source of vitamin C the year round was found in animal organs. (Muscle meats were fed to the dogs or huskies which pulled the Eskimo sleds.)

Stef said that as a result of this diet there was no disease among the Eskimos: no scurvy, arthritis, diabetes, tooth decay, or even cancer. Recent scare stories have appeared in various publications insisting that the high amount of fat in any diet is a cause of breast cancer. According to sound anthropological research[2] cancer was NOT evident in the Eskimos, or other primitive tribes on similar diets. Stef reported that the Eskimos were completely free of cancer *until* the offering of processed foods of the white man became available through the trading posts.[2] Then, and then only, for the first time, did cancer appear, as well as other common ailments.

Meanwhile Stefansson was being criticized by American "experts" who said that the reason the Eskimo diet worked for that tribe was because they lived in a cold climate. Stefansson, who was normally gentle, became infuriated at this false conclusion and offered himself, and a companion, Karsten Anderson, who had also spent time in the Arctic, as human guinea pigs to be studied by Bellevue Hospital in New York City to prove that the diet would work in any climate. The offer was accepted and the study lasted for nearly a year through the varying climates of the eastern United States, including the hot, humid summer. The two men expected to be followed by spies who believed they would cheat at every opportunity, sneak a candy bar or other carbohydrate food not in the Eskimo diet. The two men were right; the spies were evident and even followed them into telephone booths, trying to catch them cheating on the diet. Stef told me, "What they could not understand is that when you are on this diet, you neither get hungry nor crave carbohydrates!" I also found this true, while I was on the diet.

Stef and Anderson were given every possible medical test before and after the extensive study and nearly a year later on the diet, were found to still be in perfect health. In spite of the high fat intake, cholesterol proved normal. Also there was no artery and no heart trouble. Nobody could believe it. The study made international history. The "experts" had to surrender!

The next step was taken by A. W. Pennington, M.D., a company doctor for the E.I. Dupont de Nemours plant in Wilmington, Delaware, called the Du Pont Company. Dr. Pennington enlisted overweight Du Pont volunteers, of whom there were many. Again, medical tests were given before and after. Apparently there was a company cafeteria on the premises. The volunteers were asked to take a thirty minute walk before breakfast, probably to increase circulation, although Blake Donaldson, M.D., the doctor who had used the diet successfully with his patients, has stated that during a thirty minute pre-breakfast walk, within the first ten minutes the bile begins to drain from the liver and gallbladder, and in the last twenty minutes one can expect a pint of bile to drain off, carrying away a tremendous overnight waste from the body.[1]

Following the thirty minute walk at Du Pont the employees returned to a breakfast of meat and fat with no toast, no cereals or other carbohydrates. Favorites were pork chops or lamp chops, broiled without trimming the fat. Or if a leaner hamburger patty or steak were served, a pat of butter was placed on top for additional fat. At the end of the six week study, tests showed the volunteers in excellent health. Furthermore, all had lost weight.[3]

Stefansson himself, when eating at a restaurant, where my husband and I often joined Stef and his lovely wife, Eve, usually ordered rare roast beef. He gave the waiter strict instructions for the chef not to trim off the fat!

Obviously, those who enjoy fat enjoy this diet. Others often learn to enjoy it. But those who can't are the exceptions, of course.

Does one miss bread or sugar? After I had been on the diet and thrived on it I must confess I became gradually lazy and returned to bread with butter, which I later realized is an addiction.

This diet was originally called the Stefansson Diet, but later, after it was first reported in the old *Holiday* magazine, it became known as the "Holiday Diet," a misnomer, since it implied to some people that it was restricted to holidays. It was later changed to the Du Pont

Diet. I still prefer to call it the Stefansson diet, since it was discovered by Stefansson.

With those who believe the Eskimos were a fat race, Stefansson disagreed. He said that as he lived with them in their igloos he saw them stripped of clothes and they were not only healthy, but lean. Their clothes and their short, somewhat stocky build when covered with heavy furs merely gave the false impression of fat.

Please keep in mind that copious research agrees from medical doctors as well as anthropologists (whose business it is to note the effects of civilization on man) that the Eskimos living on their original *native* primitive diet remained healthy until the trading posts appeared, offering civilized foods such as canned vegetables, sugar, white flour products, and alcohol. According to Dr. Price when the tribes became addicted to these "new foods," only then did their disease rate, including cancer, begin to soar. Some writers have insisted that these tribes like the Hunzas remained well because they ate very little meat. Today's anthropologists deny this. As spokesman Leon Abrams, Jr., an Associate Professor of Anthropology, University Systems of Georgia, explains, the native tribes actually preferred protein, but only when they could not get it in sufficient amounts did they turn to vegetables because they became hungry.

Agricultural tests show that the grains and cereals being grown today, as well as vegetables, are gradually becoming lower in protein. The late Dr. W. A. Albrecht, Dean Emeritus, Department of Soils, College of Agriculture, University of Missouri, found that animal malnutrition as well as human malnutrition was due to overcropped, infertile soil. Exact figures showed that the greatest number of draft rejectees in World War II came from areas where soils were the poorest.[4]

Anthropologist Leon Abrams also has revealed that good health is greater where more protein was available to help body cells (also made of protein) repair themselves with foods rich in the protein amino acids. His research shows that over the centuries, vegetarianism was *not* the food of the healthiest populations. Dr. Price agreed with this premise as he evaluated his fourteen primitive tribes. Even vegetables raised on a high mineral soil (hard to find today) were used only as a last resort, and as a result in some countries, vegetarianism produced a higher death rate at an earlier age. India is one example.

Tests in this country show that corn is annually diminishing rapidly in protein content and other grains and plants are following suit. Whole grains including whole wheat are also deteriorating, as well as being refined in addition to the fact, as mentioned ealier, that wheat is now considered the number one allergen in this country by a major medical clinic. Thousands of people are allergic to it, without realizing it.

Protein is apparently needed for health. The fat added to it to increase its "assimilation" and other benefits is a more recent finding by Stefansson and associates. So the basis of the Stefansson diet is a high intake fat-protein with no carbohydrates (i.e. anything made of sugar or flour). If you feel you *must* have some carbohydrates, even the whole cereal or grains or bread made from them, it is considered safe in this diet to eat them providing you eat them *alone* at a separate meal, not in connection with proteins and fats. Those who argue that fats are high in calories are correct. But research shows that the fat helps to "burn" or assimilate the protein in the diet as well as remove excess fat in the body.

Many reports show that this fat/protein combination helps to streamline the body as well as the arteries. Some of the newest research on cholesterol control shows that taking carbohydrates with fat (even bread with butter) can produce the "gluey" substance which clogs the arteries. So the recent research based on extensive tests, tends to show that cholesterol is due, not to the *fat* intake, as previously thought, but to *carbohydrates,* especially when combined with fats. This apparently explains why those tribes living on this primitive diet were free of artery and heart disease. You will have to prove this to yourself. Only when you find that you can climb stairs without huffing and puffing, and begin to experience that "top of the world feeling" will you believe this. Mixing fats with carbohydrates, however, will not bring good results.

Isn't it interesting and somewhat suspicious that books written by medical physicians extolling this diet and followed in every case with thousands of unsolicited testimonials of health improvement, have suddenly become obliterated? Since this diet is based on the "uncivilized diet'' regardless of the tribe, could it be that those who are try-ing to ''sell'' us on civilized foods for their own benefit have blocked the sale of books telling the other side of the story? Today, of the many books written about the success of the diet, almost the only re-maining one I could find in print is that of Robert Atkins, also an M.D., who has applied the diet mainly to weight reduction.[5] And judging by his statements in his books, the road has not been easy for him. He has apparently been blocked at every turn, while the public is widely enthusiastic not only about their weight loss without hunger, but the other good health effects, as a sort of bonus. Dr. Atkins also recommends vitamins (which does not make him pop-ular with nonnutritional doctors).

HOW TO USE THIS DIET

There are many people who will pooh-pooh this diet, insisting that it is normal to be able to eat anything and everything, and that re-stricted combinations are not natural. I once thought this myself. But today it is hard to find a so-called ''normal'' person. We have al-ready discovered that metabolisms vary from person to person. In addition, nearly everyone has an allergy of some kind, and almost everyone is said to have hypoglycemia. Countless people also com-plain of fatigue, colds, headaches, sinus, overweight, insomnia and a plethora of other ailments. If you are one of these, then doctors who have used this diet in their practice so successfully, recommend the version of this diet, called the ''Curative Diet.'' This means that at first you follow the diet *exactly* without cheating. Then as you be-gin to recover, the doctors assure you that you can gradually add more carbohydrates until you reach your own metabolic level, mean-ing whatever agrees with you and then you may adhere to it as a maintenance diet.

I will not take up valuable space here to enumerate the names of the many physicians who report health successes with this type of diet, but I will list some of the ailments they have reported which they have seen greatly improved or even reversed by use of the diet:

Allergies	Arthritis	Fatigue: lack of
Artery & heart	Depression	vitality
problems	Diabetes	Frequent colds

Gas (flatulence)	Indigestion	Obesity
Gall bladder	High cholesterol	a host of other
disturbance	Hypoglycemia	ailments

For laymen or physicians who read this list and refuse to accept it, considering it "Unscientific," let me remind them that this list was not compiled by me, merely reported by M.D.'s who had achieved success with patients who suffered from such ailments. Their experiences and tests have convinced them, though they, too, at first were skeptical. And, again, it may not work for everyone. This diet should not be evaluated without a try, at least! Hundreds of thousands have attested to its success, which should mean something. One explanation why this diet works is that the protein apparently helps to reactivate and rehabilitate cells so that the body heals itself, while the fat activates the protein.

It is important that this diet, used today, include uncontaminated animal protein, which the public should demand. Quality of food is probably more important than quantity.

The Stefansson diet used with no substitutes by doctors who prescribed it for health purposes, was called the "Curative Diet." It is as follows:

RULES FOR THE CURATIVE DIET

1. Eat a complete assortment of natural foods of all types: meat, fats, vegetables (as many raw as possible); fruits in moderation (due to sugar content), in order to get a full varied supply of vitamins and minerals as provided by Nature. The Orientals are said to eat thirty or more different foods daily; Americans seem to be limited to about sixteen.[6]

2. Avoid processed sugar in any form as well as processed food, which means nutrients have been removed, and additives probably included.

3. Eat fats freely with proteins, but do not eat high proteins (meat, fish, eggs, cheese) with high starches of any kind. (List of starches follows on page . . .).

4. Use acids with proteins, but not with starches. (Proteins need acid for digestion; starches do not.)

5. Use meat, fish, eggs, dairy products once or more daily with

fats. Sour cream, butter, and whipped cream used with proteins are acceptable for fat, as are some natural oils such as olive oil which is a fruit oil (not made from seeds). Since oils are often processed with chemicals or excessive heat it is better to take oily seeds: i.e. for almond oil, eat almonds; for peanut oil eat peanuts; for sunflower oil, eat sunflower seeds. When the industry learns to make or press oils naturally, then the oils will be more healthful and nutritious. Fish liver oils are excellent.

6. Eat fruits and green and yellow vegetables, raw if possible: two servings daily or one large salad bowl full (recipe follows).

7. Eat cereals or so-called whole grains if you are not intolerant to them, at a *separate* meal. Do not combine with fats or acids. (Most whole grains today are deficient. Refining removes 60-80% of vitamins and minerals in wheat and 87% of the bran or fiber.)[6]

8. Use vitamin/mineral supplements for your special needs.

HOW LONG WILL IT TAKE

How long will it take to see results? Doctors agree that your own health condition as well as your age are factors to consider. The younger, the better. The results in some people are conditioned by their past eating habits. Daniel Munro, M.D., wrote in his out-of-print book, *Man Alive You're Half Dead*[9] "If you now suffer from occasional gas, a month or more on the regimen with no cheating will work wonders. If you feel OK yet sluggish and under par and have been eating unwisely of breads, cakes, desserts and such, on the new regimen you should begin to experience a feeling of well-being you may not have believed possible."

Dr. Munro recommends a protein-and-fat meal twice daily— perhaps at breakfast and dinner, and the following sumptuous salad at lunch:

BOUNTIFUL SALAD (A whole meal lunch)

In an aged and fragrant wooden salad bowl, combine:
- small sections of lettuce, watercress, romaine or spinach
- raw shredded root vegetables such as carrots, beets, celery, plus

raw onion rings or geen onions chopped, green peppers, radishes, sprouts, avocado, raw peas, summer squash, sliced cucumbers, raw potatoes, or whatever is in season and *fresh*, preferably right out of your own garden. Use your ingenuity. Add thin slivers of cheese, cold meat, chicken, or small balls of cottage cheese, or sliced hard boiled egg.

Top with virgin (unrefined) olive oil, sprinkle with fresh lemon juice, or garlic flavored or plain wine vinegar. Season with the whole or herb salt, perhaps fresh ground pepper, or if possible, add garden herbs cut fine: parsley, basil, thyme and any others available. Toss well and serve.

No bread, toast, crackers, sweets or other high carbohydrates are used here. You have a balanced selection of vitamins, minerals, fiber. Since the water content is high, little beverage is needed. Plain, *un*sweetened yogurt may be used as "a dessert." This salad alone makes a yummy and satisfying lunch. As Dr. Atkins says, if you are on a serious reducing diet, your days of bread, sugar and sugar products are over forever! Perhaps those who are prone to cholesterol, heart or artery problems should follow suit. How will you manage without them? Dr. Munro answers, "At first I found this strange. After the habit was broken, I enjoyed my food more than ever."

MEAL PLANNING TIPS

Breakfast—Eggs with natural bacon (no nitrates) plus butter, or natural sausage, (read labels) or an omelet. Juice may be served with this protein breakfast *if* it is an acid-type (citrus if you can tolerate it) or tomato juice. (No sweet juices). Sauteed tomatoes or mushrooms may be added. Or you may make a Spanish omelet from eggs, chopped onions, tomatoes, green pepper or an omelet of lightly sauteed or raw mushrooms. Adding a bit of onion contributes flavor.

You may prefer a carbohydrate breakfast, consisting of a whole sweet fruit (no citrus) plus a "whole grain" cereal, with milk, *no cream,* plus a tiny bit of honey if absolutely necessary. Use toast or bread or crackers, but *no butter.*

Lunch—salad as described, or meat with fat of some kind, (no cottage cheese salad with fruit unless acid fruit.) If you wish a carbohydrate type of lunch, you can use high starch vegetables, such as potatoes, (but no butter). Those who have tried it insist that a baked potato with salt and pepper is highly edible. Or you may have spaghetti, or baked beans and any high starchy vegetable. Whole, non-acid fruit or dessert is OK here.

Dinner can be a duplicate of breakfast, or contain dairy products, chops, or roast, or fowl or liver and bacon. A low starch vegetable or a small salad can be added to any protein meal. Dry wine is permissible with your protein meal, if used in moderation, say a 4 oz. glass.

What about sandwiches? How can you make them without bread? I have licked this one by using thin slices of cheese. I often put cucumber slices, chopped onion and mayonnaise or a protein type filling between the two thin cheese slices. Good and satisfying. Or use lettuce leaves for enclosing gooey mixtures such as you might add to tacos - green peppers, shredded lettuce, tomatoes, sprouts, grated cheese, chopped meat, mayonnaise, etc. Good. Various doctors have added their own ideas, which may or may not be advisable. One doctor allowed a demitasse (a half cup) of coffee with each meal. Although it is true that hypoglycemia (hyper-insulinism) seems to disappear on this diet, feel your way cautiously with coffee. It still may not be for you. Another doctor warned against drinking water with meals, particularly protein meals, for fear of diluting HCl (hydrochloric acid) needed for protein digestion. Newer research suggests that it is better to sip water if you need it and take HCl as a supplement after protein meals. Some people never have sufficient HCl, otherwise.

Another observation of caution: When this diet first began to be published, vitamin therapy was not only new, but certainly not taught to M.D.'s in medical school (it still isn't). Therefore the doctors who felt that vitamins were necessary had to learn their way alone. Since then knowledge about vitamins has come a long way and you may find you know more about, or can find out more solid information about vitamin therapy than the doctors. Some of them have not yet recognized minerals: one doctor mistakenly calls the mineral calcium, a "vitamin." The best sources of all-natural mineral combinations from ancient deep sea beds being used today by nutrition-conscious physicians are *Minerals 72*[7] and *Azomite,*[8] both in powder or tablet form. Great results have occurred by the consistent use of these natural minerals. (Azomite also contains a volcanic ash derivative).

SIDE EFFECTS OF THE DIET

Are there any side effects of this diet? Yes, but they are only temporary. In the first week, constipation is common, usually tapering off during the second week. A natural herbal laxative may help some (not others), or a tablespoon of flax seed (followed with water) or psyllium seed night and morning taken in water; or even better as mentioned earlier, a fiber product to provide bulk which helps nearly everyone. One brand is called *Fy-Blend* and is available in health stores. Another, called *Intestinal Cleanser,* is available from Price Pottenger Nutrition Foundation. P.O. Box 2116, La Mesa, Ca 92041. You take a tablespoon of the fiber product or a teaspoon of the Intestinal Cleanser in water morning and night and stir, then swallow quickly before it becomes too thick to swallow. Follow with more water.

The second side effect of the diet occurs during the first two or three weeks: the diet acts as a diuretic. People who are trying to lose weight will be overjoyed, but hear this: Any diuretic washes B vitamins out of the body, together with essential minerals. Extra amounts of both should be taken to compensate. So do not worry if your kidneys keep you running to the bathroom. But do keep up your intake of the disappearing B vitamins and minerals to compensate for any loss! The condition will eventually cease.

The Stefansson diet calls for protein plus fat, though low starch foods (5% - 10%) are allowed.

QUESTIONS AND ANSWERS

Q. What do I do if I do not want to lose weight, but gain it?

A. As I suggested, read Dr. Atkins' *Super-Energy* book. He has worked out all the fine points for both finding

HIGH AND LOW STARCHES

Low starch fruits and vegetables are those in the 5% and 10% lists. The high starches are those in the 15% and 20% lists.

LOW STARCHES	HIGH STARCHES

5% VEGETABLES

Asparagus	Greens	Radishes
Bean sprouts	Kohlrabi	Rhubarb
Brussels sprouts	Leeks	Sauerkraut
Cabbage	Lettuce	Spinach
Cauliflower	Mushrooms	String beans
Celery	Okra	Summer squash
Cucumbers	Olives	Swiss chard
Eggplant	Peppers	Tomatoes
Endive	Pumpkin	Watercress

FRUITS

Lemon juice	Watermelon
Honeydew melon	Muskmelon
Rhubarb	

15% VEGETABLES

Lima beans (young)
Parsnips
Peas

FRUITS

Apples
Apricots
Blueberries
Cherries (sour)
Grapes
Loganberries
Mulberries
Pears
Pineapples
Pineapple juice
Plums
Raspberries

These foods may be used with protein meals in the dietary.

10% VEGETABLES

Beets	Oyster plant	Squash
Carrots	Rutabagas	Turnips
Onions		

FRUITS

Blackberries	Gooseberries	Orange juice
Cranberries	Grapefruit	Peaches
Currants	Lime juice	Strawberries

(acceptable with protein)

These foods acceptable with the 5% low starch foods above with protein meals in the dietary.

20% VEGETABLES

Beans
  Kidney
  Lima
  Navy
Corn
Macaroni
Bananas
Grape juice
Cherries, sweet

Bread is a high starch food.

Chart by Daniel C. Munro, M.D.

your own best maintenance diet as well as one for gaining weight, or acquiring more energy. Space is limited here. His book is available at any book store in paperback. You will find it excellent.

Q.   What about using black pepper? Most nutritionists claim it is a no-no.
A.   This is a partial story only. A diet system in India called "Tridosha" states that black pepper is one of our best foods if it is freshly ground from peppercorns as needed. Once ground, however, it becomes rancid when stored in bottles or cans and is *un*wholesome.

Q.   I hate cod-liver oil. Is there any easy way to take it?
A.   I hate it too, but there is a pleasant way to take it as suggested by Dale Alexander, the cod liver oil specialist. He suggests taking one tablespoon of mint-flavored cod liver oil (from drug or health stores) and adding it ice-cold to a small amount of ice cold orange juice, or other juice, if you are allergic to orange. I keep a small jar which formerly contained olives, or pimentos, etc. and combine the oil and juice in it, and drink from the jar. I do not wash it with the rest of the dishes since it spreads the odor to them. When its use is over, I throw the jar away and use another. The flavor of this combination is delightful. Taken first thing in the morning or last thing at night on an empty stomach (to avoid weight gain) it is truly palatable.

Q.   Isn't the Stefansson diet expensive in these times?
A.   Unfortunately yes. Dr. Atkins says it is a luxury diet, but he adds that since one is not hungry on the diet, less food is used overall, whereas carbohydrates diets usually make you ravenous for more.

My own reaction is that health at any price is *cheap*. When your car wears out you can buy a new one (also at a price these days). You cannot buy a new body, at any price. At our house, we would rather pay the butcher or the health store than the hospital, or other types of questionable non-nutritional medical care or drugs, which are also expensive, perhaps less effective in many cases, and also less comfortable.

SOME CASE REPORTS

Now for some case reports from doctors who *have* used this primitive diet on their patients.

Dr. Daniel C. Munro starts with himself. He writes[9] "Following these principles I find that I can now accomplish physical exertions which were formerly impossible such as skiing, mountain climbing as well as sports requiring speed and fast reaction time." The following cases are actual and true experiences of his patients:

One woman was a victim of colitis and arthritis, and had tried "everything." Dr. Munro put her on the diet plus vitamins A, D, and B complex. Weeks later her pain was gone and she looked years younger.

A banker also complained of his arthritis as well as an acid stomach with resulting pain. He had given up golf as a result. He also suffered from insomnia. Dr. Munro believed he had a complete deficiency of vitamin C and added it to the primitive diet as well as tomato juice. The banker insisted the tomato juice would irritate his "acid stomach." The doctor told him it would not if he took it only with the protein meals. In due time his stomach distress disappeared, he was sleeping soundly, awoke each morning feeling better than he had for months. He returned to his golf.

Another doctor, a colleague, asked for a complete physical examination, appearing somewhat smug as well as fearful because he had no disease but anticipated it anyway. Dr. Munro pointed out that he already had severe dental problems and receding gums, and the more serious disease could follow. This man was on a "civilized" diet and a changeover to the Stefansson "uncivilized" type diet surprised him by bringing general health improvement as well as prevention of the disease he was fearing.

Another man with plenty of leisure and money to indulge himself in expensive health spas prided himself on not eating any animal products. He was a strict vegetarian, and according to Dr. Munro's tests, on the verge of a complete collapse. He suffered from edema, high blood pressure and general exhaustion. At first, the patient refused to eat protein. He finally agreed to give the diet a try as he felt so bad, and Dr. Munro said that as a result, his health not only became good; he looked more attractive.

Another Munro case was that of a hospitalized banker with serious gall bladder trouble whose chance of living was doubtful. He insisted he didn't have time to think about food. Dr. Munro put him on his bountiful lunch salad as well as the rest of "the diet." The man who had left the hospital where X-rays showed a diseased intestinal tract finally agreed to eat the "rabbit food" as well as the rest of the diet. He found he enjoyed it and a year later he said he felt fine, could now play golf and his friends agreed that he looked better and healthier than he had for years, according to Dr. Munro.

Blake Donaldson, M.D., in his book, *Strong Medicine*[1] describes many cases of success of his use of the primitive diet, together with other measures, such as weight loss and exercise. He is perhaps the most orthodox of all doctors who have written on this subject, and did not use vitamins. But with the diet as a basis of his work, he achieved some remarkable results. The case histories are too detailed and long to include here but he made some wise statements along the way in his book:

p. 107: "Flour and sugar are too rich for most of us and are only usable for those who do heavy manual labor."

p. 122: on high blood pressure: "You will do better working than loafing, with high blood pressure."

p. 113: on arteriosclerosis: "Lack of regular outdoor exercise is one possible cause of arteriosclerosis."

p. 32: on nutrition and teeth: "Cells may have common needs in nutrition. The best foods to prevent cataracts in the eyes and holes in the teeth may also treat migraine, duodenal ulcer and heart disease."

"The teeth are always the easiest system in the human body to study."

p. 35: "In this country the real deficiency state is not due to a lack of vitamins, but to a lack of amino acids. We must get enough of these essential amino acids to keep our body cells in a state of good repair . . . therefore from what I have observed, a half pound of meat per meal is the minimum quantity needed to maintain the work of the body cells.''

p. 33: on fat: "The primitive peoples seemed to crave fat if they could get it.''

p. 35: "Fat in itself is not well-digested alone. It must be mixed with something else. When combined with meat, "trial and error seems to show that today a good fat/meat ratio is about three parts of fat to one of meat.''

p. 130: on energy: "Those on this [primitive] diet comment on the sudden development of well being, often within three days. That should be due to the increased amino acids but no one can be sure.'' (Others believe it is the fat/protein combination.)

Dr. Donaldson was a bit more lenient in his version of the primitive diet, allowing some butter on potatoes, since he considered potatoes not a starchy root but a "stem" vegetable. He was also the one to allow a demitasse of coffee with each meal.

HOW ABOUT TODAY'S FOODS VS. THOSE OF THE PRIMITIVES?

Let's face our present day civilization. Due to contamination of air and water, and contamination as well as depletion of soil on which our plants are raised, plus the many additives, pesticides and hormones in not only carbohydrate foods, but in meats and fats, our food is far different from those plants, or protein foods (fish and meat) as well as fats, used by the primitives. What are we to do? The public must *demand* safe food so that such primitive diets as the Stefansson diet are safe to eat. We can only expect food reforms if we are relentless, good consumers, demanding the best, not half-way measures. As long as we put up with less than the best we will receive it. We must hold fast in our insistence on *the best*.

Many people are beginning to worry about this and are also beginning to do something about it. They are raising their own foods, and, if they are unable to raise their safe dairy products, fowl and food animals, are looking for someone who can.

In the next chapter I will describe one country which has developed near perfect food, and I will tell you what one American family, thoroughly knowledgeable about the Price primitive diets, eats for health today.

NOTES

1. Blake F. Donaldson, M.D., *Strong Medicine.* New York: Doubleday, 1962.

2. Vilhjalmur Stefansson, *Cancer: Disease of Civilization?* New York: Hill and Wang (?), 1960.

3. A. W. Pennington, "Treatment of Obesity with Calorically Unrestricted Diets." *Journal of Clinical Nutrition* 1:100, 1953.

4. *Geographical Review,* Vol. 47, 1957, pages 86-105.

5. Robert Atkins, M.D., *Dr. Atkins' Diet Revolution.* New York: Bantam, 1973. Paperback.

Robert Atkins, M.D., with Shirley Linde, *Dr. Atkins' Superenergy Diet.* New York: Bantam, 1978. Paperback.

6. Charles T. McGee, M.D., *How To Survive Modern Technology.* Alamo, CA: Ecology Press, 1979.

7. For information on Minerals 72, ask health stores or write: Beauty Naturally, Inc. P.O. Box 426, Fairfax, CA 94930, enclosing stamp or letter size self-addressed stamped envelope.

8. For Azomite write Azone, Utah Mining Co., Sterling, Utah, 84665, enclosing self-addressed stamped envelope.

9. Daniel C. Monro, M.D., *Man Alive You're Half Dead.* New York: Bartholomew House, 1940. This book is out of print.

CHAPTER FIFTEEN

How to Eat Well in a Declining World

A friend called me as I was about to close this book and I was so inspired by what she told me I decided to share the information with you. Kay and her husband, a retired college art professor, had just returned from a trip to France. He was interested in art museums, ancient castles and other architecture. Kay merely accompanied him for companionship. She, however, is a great cook and extremely food-conscious as well as quick about learning good nutrition. This particular tour was on a barge which was engine-driven on a canal through French wine and farm country during the daytime, and anchored offshore at night. From time to time it halted at various villages or other spots of interest. At that time, the French cook, a young woman, would go ashore to do her shopping for the three daily meals served the passengers on board the barge. And what meals!

On these shopping expeditions, the cook would return to the barge laden with freshly picked farm produce as well as fresh dairy products. The farm houses were small and humble, but each one was surrounded with a huge, neat and meticulously cared for garden. Fruits and berries were homegrown as well as vegetables of all varieties. Nothing was thrown away. All kitchen scraps were composted and added to the soil, and since each farm had its own animals, chickens, goats, rabbits and cows, manure was added liberally. The soil was not allowed to become depleted and as the barge passed these farms, the women were seen doing the work of adding the natural fertilizers as well as weeding and caring for the garden in general. They did it not as a chore, but lovingly and proudly (it is also good exercise). Kay learned that chemical fertilizers were shunned and insecticide sprays were not necessary or used. There were no contaminating factories allowed in the area and the air, the soil and the water were not contaminated. Since there was no run-off of dangerous chemicals from the gardens into nearby streams and rivers, fresh fish caught there were safe and delicious. Eggs were fertile since the chickens (hens and roosters) were allowed to run naturally on the ground.

Dairy products were taken from cows which grazed on green fields, visible for miles around. The butter, served sweet (unsalted), was a natural lemon yellow color rather than colored artifically; and was soft, melting easily at room or body temperature as it should be. On the barge, it was served in rolls, then sliced into individual servings and placed in a butter dish, one on each table. Cream was thick and rich, cheese varied and delicious. On a plate of assorted cheeses served for dessert were small flags identifying each variety.

Meat and fowl were raised without chemicals, Kay learned. She was not given much information about flour, although it, too, was obviously homegrown on good soil. The famous crusty French bread, fresh from the bakery, was served daily and the warm croissants bought fresh just before breakfast by a boy sent to shore before the barge started its daily journey, were mouth watering, (served of course with the sweet butter) as anyone knows who has tried them.

I asked Kay to describe the menus in general.

Breakfast was the usual continental breakfast, either with tea or cafe-au-lait (half and half coffee and hot milk, raw, natural and unpasteurized from the farms). Bowls of whole homegrown fruit were also served with the croissants.

Lunch consisted of an assortment of from five to seven different salads, including every available type of fresh raw garden vegetable. Many were sliced, others such as beets and carrots, grated. A simple French dressing of fragrant oil (the French often use virgin—the first pressing—olive oil, when available) plus wine vinegar, a bit of salt (whole salt is available in France) and finely minced garden herbs of many kinds, sprinkled over the whole salad bowl before tossing.

Occasionally, at lunch, there were cheese and egg dishes such as quiche (a type of one-crust savory pie). Soups were made of *whole* vegetables: thick, not thin.

Dinner consisted of a protein straight from the farm, plus salads and/or fresh vegetables, lightly cooked. Occasionally, for dessert instead of the assorted cheese, tarts made from the native fruit were served. Since this was wine country, wine was also served.

Kay says she has never eaten such delicious food, not only due to expert cooking, but mainly due to the excellent quality and flavor, a result of good soil management.

Kay confessed that she could hardly wait from one meal to the next. I asked her if she put on weight. She said no, she lost two pounds. She admitted that this was partly due to extensive walking (everyone else rode bicycles) since she was eager to visit the French housewives and observe the gardens at close range. The women were healthy, happy and contented, a fact often noted in other well-nourished communities.

Kay, herself, said that she had left the United States exhausted after a busier than usual schedule before departing. Yet, she added, that as a result of that natural countryside and the excellent food she returned home feeling better than ever.

If France can do this, why not America?

AN AMERICAN FAMILY'S EATING PLAN

Let me introduce to you a family which uses the information provided in Dr. Price's book, *Nutrition and Physical Degeneration*. This family has set as their goal a determination to live in these times, on a diet as close as possible to the quality of the primitive foods discovered and studied by Dr. Price.

The members of the family include the wife, the husband, Joe, a nutritionally oriented dentist, who applies the information not only to his own diet, but to his patients as well, with great success; two grown boys including a son and a friend, whose status in the family is similar to that of an exchange student. He is newer to the nutritional approach than the others, but is eager and learning fast.

The husband, Dr. Joseph Connolly, is a nutritionally oriented dentist, who applies the information not only to his own diet, but to his patients as well, with great success.

There are two grown boys in the family, a son, Joe III, and Willie, whose status in the family is similar to that of an exchange student.

He is newer to the nutritional approach than the others, but is eager and learning fast.

Each member of the family eats a slightly different diet, yet in harmony with the whole primitive concept, though individually adjusted to the personal tastes and needs of each. Even though the diets may have varied over the years, the goal remains the same: to try to achieve primitive quality food. Though they live in a city they try to grow as much of their raw salad material and vegetables as possible, using the French Intensive Bio-Dynamic techniques in spite of certain restrictions on their city lot. They compost their vegetables wastes, and also add to their garden soil seaweed plus rock materials and Azomite, a mineral combination derived from an ancient seabed.

For drinking water, to bypass city water, they use a distiller, later adding Azomite to replace the missing minerals removed by distilling. They feel that they are doing the best they can in spite of a polluted environment and polluted air. And they do far more than most Americans.

Here are some of their choices.

Breakfast

They soak one or more of the following seeds for twenty-four hours in pure water: sunflower, flax, sesame, chia, pumpkin or other seeds. The boys use two tablespoons of each. The boys sometimes add fruit, such as a chopped apple or other fruit cut into bite size. Willie adds pineapple juice to his "seed cereal" whereas the rest of the family add cream or their cream substitute which they make and call "fake" cream.*

The father admits that he will eat anything if it is good for him. The wife and the boys believe they digest their food better if it tastes good as well. The father grinds his seeds (unsoaked) and adds milk or water or cream.

Sometimes the mother serves one of the several whole grains instead of seeds for the morning cereal. In a covered pan, she places

---

*Recipe is available in *Guide to Living Foods*—Price-Pottenger Nutrition Foundation, P.O. Box 1624, La Mesa, CA 92041

millet, rye, brown rice, barley, whole oats, etc. and water, bringing them to a boil and then turning off the heat, allowing the grains to steam and remain in the covered pan overnight. In the morning the consistency is perfect.

This family formerly used various natural flavorings or sweeteners, such as honey, carob, butter, sea salt, fruit for flavor, even date sugar. They have given up this habit, which they believe is unnecessary, partly because they are trying to wean themselves of the sweet and salt addictions, and partly because the wife is on the Stefansson curative diet at the present time and this outlaws sweets taken with protein, which is said to interfere with protein digestion.

Occasionally for variation, this family makes egg nogs from fertile eggs and goat's milk or fake cream. Also, occasionally, they buy frozen brains cut into chunks to add raw to the eggnog (or put in the blender). This drink is because the boys demand it at exam times. Joe III is trying to get into medical school; Willie aspires to dental school and both boys say they *know* from experience that the "brain nog" helps their memory recall during exams. At other times the whole family eats for breakfast liver, or lamb kidneys, sometimes raw, cut into small pieces, or lightly broiled. (Both are acceptable on the Curative Diet.)

The favorite beverage is chicory tea, bought ground and roasted. They make all herb teas by putting the herb in a bottle of cold water and placing it in the refrigerator to soak. They use 9 teaspoons of chicory per half gallon of water. It is served cold or hot, with or without cream. Other herb tea favorites are red clover, pink lemon, raspberry, Kaf-free and others from Sunshine Valley available at health stores. They do not eat fried eggs, ham, bacon, sausage, toast, jam or even granola for breakfast since they want *fresh* food, raw when possible.

SNACKS

If snacks are desired, though the family usually does not get hungry midmorning, they use one of several varieties of nuts: macadamia, Brazil, pistachio, pecans, almonds and sunflower and pumpkin seeds. The nuts are used straight from the shells, cracked and chewed well; the seeds are pre-hulled for convenience.

LUNCH

If Joe III takes his lunch, it includes leftover meat or fish, or raw steak, often with soy sauce poured over it, packed in a glass jar plus half a cucumber, some cherry tomatoes, celery, carrots or Jerusalem artichokes, (all raw of course). Or sometimes the mother makes these ingredients plus leftover protein into a salad with homemade mayonnaise, homemade dill pickles also packed in a glass jar. Those eating at home have a *large* raw vegetable salad with sprouts and any leftover dinner fish or meat, added in slivers. The salad dressing varies from anchovy, guacamole, Piima[1], herbs or chia seed dressings. Pat begins her salad dressings with olive oil plus a splash of garlic vinegar or lemon juice. If no salad is used, there is a platter of raw vegetables on the table, including raw broccoli, carrots, peppers, celery, cukes, Jerusalem artichokes, cauliflower, etc., sometimes with dips. Soups include tomato shrimp, beet borscht, vegetable, lentil or split pea, enhanced by juices left from steaming yesterday's vegetables, usually served at dinner time.

DINNER

Dinner consists of organ meats whenever available: sweet breads, liver, kidney, or meat, fish or fowl often served with herb butter.[9] Steamed vegetables or a small salad finish the meal. If the boys are starved, baked potatoes or squash, kasha, millet or pinto beans help fill them up.

Yogurt or Piima* is made with goat's milk and used often and in many ways even as a garnish or sliced vegetables together with a sardine, anchovy or olive-half and Piima are used as an appetizer.

The mother is a gourmet at heart and is always investigating new foods and experimenting to see how she can make them palatable without destroying their nutrient value. There are loads of recipes she has devised, including a coconut birthday cake, homemade caviar and champagne, and others.[2]

---

*Recipes and Piima starter (similar to yogurt) available from Price-Pottenger Nutrition Foundation, Box 2116, La Mesa, CA 92041

The diet of this family may seem Spartan, but they deserve credit for refusing to be brainwashed by the food and other commercial industries. Their philosophy is that our Creator gave us natural food for perfect health whereas man has tampered with it resulting in illness.

THE DEMONSTRATION CENTER

Plans are afoot for the Price-Pottenger Nutrition Foundation to acquire land on which they can raise primitive-type food, including fish, fowl, and other safe feed animals. Helpful information on gardening methods, as well as health improvement tips will be studied and reported in the *PPNF Membership Bulletin* and the *Good Health Keeping* Newsletter.[3] Any method which can be used to preserve nutrients and protect foods and help humanity through balanced soil, pure water, clean air and good nutrition will be studied and reported along the way to help the world once again become safe for health as it was in primitive times.

Charles McGee, M.D., has stated, "Isolated primitive people remain free from degenerative diseases as long as they stay on diets of traditional unrefined foods . . . Man appears to adapt well to food as long as it is wholesome and has not been tampered with."[4]

As Dr. Royal Lee stated, the lesson to be learned is clear! "Raw, organically grown foods are our best protective foods—counterfeit foods our greatest threat! There is no substitute for live foods, no way to beat nature at her own game! The rules are set by Providence and cannot be changed, only interpreted by man's intellect. The only referee in life's battle is the Almighty!"

Perhaps all of us would be healthier if we could eat as the primitives did and as this family is trying to do. However, in order to have the correct food, the public is going to have to demand that quality food be made available to us. In an article entitled "A Quiet Way to Achieve our Wellness Goal" by Donald B. Ardell, Ph.D. are some suggestions for improving our food choices as well as our way of life.[5] Dr. Ardell favors regulations, ordinances, rules and requirements that:

• Lead to the removal of junk food vending machines from public schools, hospitals and long-term care facilities.

• Require managers of all office buildings to provide alternative food products (nonsugared, nonprocessed, nonrefined, etc.) if junk food machines are located on the premises.

• Lessen the health-denying impact of the media by inhibiting the child-directed promotion of foods high in saturated fats, cholesterol, sugar and salt.

• Increase taxes on alcohol, tobacco, and junk foods in proportion to the harmful substances within each (e.g., alcohol content, tar and nicotine, and refined sugar/preservatives), and direct the proceeds to research on them and treatment for their effects (cirrhosis of the liver, cancer, heart disease, etc.).

• Require that sugar-coated cereals, and all other products in which sugar comprises more than 20 percent of the item, be displayed in sections of supermarkets and other food stores clearly marked as "candies and other sweets." This will not prevent people from buying junk food if they really want it or believe they need it, but will help to make consumers conscious of what they are obtaining when they choose such products.

• Encourage the Federal Trade Commission to require networks to make prime time available for ads with wellness messages (in concert with the negative appeals, such as antismoking spots).

NOTES

1. *Guide to Living Foods,* Price-Pottenger Nutrition Foundation, P.O. Box 1624, La Mesa, CA 92041.

2. Recipes and Piima starter available from Price-Pottenger Nutrition Foundation, P.O. Box 2116, La Mesa, CA 92041.

3. Good Health Keeping Newsletter, Price-Pottenger Nutrition Foundation, P.O. Box 1624, La Mesa, CA 92041.

4. Donald B. Ardell, Ph.D., "A Quiet Way to Achieve Our Wellness" *Health Quarterly* Vol. 4, No. 5, published by Keats Publishing Co., New Canaan, CT 06840.

5. Charles T. McGee, M.D., *How To Survive Modern Technology.* Alamo, CA: *Ecology Press, 1979.*

and milk intolerance, 58
Flax seed, 99, 101
Flour, 155
    see also Wheat; White flour; Whole wheat
Fluorescent light (mercury vapor), 47
Folic acid (vitamin),
    and oral contraceptives, 135
    in potatoes, 83
Food dyes, 109
Foods
    choice and preparation of, 110-113
    drying of, 111
    intolerances of, 57-58, 101, 136
    nutritional variability of, 33, 37
    saving on costs of, 109-114
    seasonal choice of, 24
    see also Natural foods; Raw foods; Whole foods
Forgetfulness, 46
Fowl, 15, 76
Fredericks, Carlton, 23, 81, 92-93, 134
Freezing, 51
French Intensive Bio-Dynamic techniques, 161
Fructose, 67-68
    see also Sugars
Fruit sugar, 67-68
Fruits, 8, 21
    cooking of, 101
    in curative diet, 148-151, 161
    enzymes in, 53-54
    fiber content of, 24, 89, 92, 94-96, 99-103, 108-109
    in primitive diet, 30-31
    starch content of, 152
Fractionated foods
    see also Processing
Fungicides, 112
    mercury in, 46
    in vegetable skins, 108
Fy-Blend (brand), 102, 151

G-154 Nutrins (brand), 118
Gall bladder
    curative diet for, 147-151
Gall stones, diet for, 90, 140
Garlic
    and mercury poisoning, 46
    selenium in, 44
Gas
    see Flatulence
Genes, 5-6, 17
    see also Heredity
Glands
    and addiction, 118-120
    adrenals, 64
    liver, 17, 42
    pituitary, 17
    and protein intake, 17
    sex, 18
    thyroid, 17, 43, 70
    see also Kidneys; Pancreas

Glucose, 122
Glucose tolerance, 42
    see also Hypoglycemia
Glutamine (brand), 119
Glutamine, 119-120
Glutathione, 46
Gluten intolerance, 57
Goat's milk, 58, 163
Good Health Keeping, 107-110, 164
Gooseberries, 152
Gout, and lead poisoning, 46
Government regulation, 62-63
    proposals for, 165
Grains, protein in, 144-145
    see also Cereals; Whole grains
Grapefruit, 100, 152
Grapes, 152
Great Nutrition Robbery, The (Hunter), 10, 92
Greens, 152
    see also Lettuce; Salads
Growth factors, 16
Guide to Fiber in Foods (Kraus), 90
Guide to Living Foods (Price-Pottenger Nutrition Foundation), 36, 56

Hair, loss of, 40, 42, 44
    nutrition of, 18, 75
    testing of, 48, 137
Handbook of Natural Remedies for Common Ailments (Clark), 118
Harper, Harold, 91-92
Hawkins, David, 105
Hay fever symptoms
    from food additives, 9
    honey and, 69
Headaches
    curative diet for, 141-142, 146-151
    and food additives, 9
    and healing process, 79
    and mercury poisoning, 46
    and oil in diet, 19-20
    and red wine, 78
    and sugar intake, 123
Healing
    honey and, 70-71
    and protein deficiency, 17
    zinc and, 42
"Healing crisis," 79
Health
    genetic and nutritional factors of, 5-6
Health Food Retailing, 75, 127
Health secret, 140-157
Heart
    nutrition of, 6, 8-9, 17
    stimulants to, 69
Heart attack
    and cadmium, 47
    and iodine, 43
    and smoking, 126, 128
    and vitamin E, 6

Heart disease
    curative diet for, 140, 146-151, 155
    Factor X in, 78
    and magnesium deficiency, 40
Heat
    and honey processing, 72
    and nutritional elements, 16
    and oil processing, 76
    see also Cooking
"Heat stroke," 64
Heavy metals, 45-48
    and criminal activity, 137
Hebrides tribes, diet of, 30
Hemicellulose fiber, 100-102
Hemoglobin, 17
Hemolasses (brand), 41
Hemorrhoids, and fiber, 90, 95
Hepar Sulph 6x, 47
Herb salt, 63
Herbal laxative, 151
Herbal teas, 124, 162
Heredity
    and alcoholism, 121
    and health, 26
    and nutritional makeup, 5-6, 12
Hiatal hernia, and fiber, 90
"Hidden hunger," 20
High power foods, 35-36
Hindhede (of Denmark), 87
Hippchen, Leonard, 106
Hippocrates, 89, 95
Hitler, Adolf, 106
Holiday Diet
    see Curative diet
Homeopathic medicines, 38, 41, 47-48, 61, 121
Honey
    benefits of, 68-70
    and cereals, 100
    contaminants in, 72-74
    healing abilities of, 69-71
    processing of, 7, 71-72
Honeydew, 152
Hormones
    as contaminants, 156
    in drugs, 61, 134-135
    and magnesium deficiency, 40
    and protein intake, 17
Howell, Edward, 51-54, 111
Huberman, Max, 127
Hungerford, Mary Jane, 105
Hunter, Beatrice Trum, 9-10, 36, 55, 72, 92
Hunza tribe, diet of, 37-38, 144
Hydrochloric acid (HCl)
    and calcium intake, 39
    and iron assimilation, 41
    and protein digestion, 19, 54
    sodium and, 64
    supplements of, 150
Hydrophilic colloids, 101-102
Hyperactivity, 105, 108

and food additives, 9
and sugar intake, 66
Hyperinsulinism, 123
see also Hypoglycemia
Hypertension
see Blood pressure
Hypoglycemia, 2, 9
and crime, 137
curative diet for, 140, 146-151
and emotional problems, 105-107
and sugar intake, 66-67, 122-123
Hypothalamus, 119-120
Hypo-thyroidism, 43

Imitation foods, 10
Indian tribes of North Canada, 30
Infection
honey and, 70
magnesium and, 40
protein deficiency and, 17
Insecticides
see Pesticides
Insomnia
and calcium deficiency, 39
curative diet for, 146-151, 154
and healing process, 79
and honey, 70
and protein intake, 16
Insulin
honey and, 71
and protein intake, 17
and sugar addiction, 123
Intestinal Cleanser (brand), 102, 151
Intestinal problems
adhesions, 101
curative diet for, 147-151
pain and cramping, 91
stenosis, 101
see also Digestion problems; Ulcers
Iodine, 43
Iodized salt, 43
Irish moss, 101
Irish people, diet of, 82
Iron, 40-41
absorption of, 91
inorganic, 61
sources of, 68, 71, 83
Iron Phosphate, 41
Irritability
and protein intake, 16-17
and sugar intake, 123
Isoleucine, 16
Isser, Joseph, 62

Joint stiffness, and honey, 70
Jones, Susan Smith, 71-72
Juices
acid, 149, 152
raw, 135
starches in, 152
Junk food, 1, 20-21, 82, 108, 120, 135, 137, 165

Karaya seeds, 101
Kelley, William Donald, 14-15, 19, 54
Kelp, for iodine, 43
see also Seafoods; Sea plants
Keyes, Elizabeth, 10
Kidneys
dysfunction of, 40
and mercury poisoning, 17
and protein intake, 17
Kirby, Rebecca, 60
Know Your Nutrition (Clark), 2, 19
Kohlrabi, 152
Kosher dill pickle, 55-56
Kosher salt, 63-64
Kouchakoff, Paul, 54-55
Kraus, Barbara, 90
Kwashiorkor, 136

Labelling
of B vitamins, 22
of fiber content, 93
of fiber supplements, 101
of foods, 9-11, 17
of honey, 72
of sugar content, 122
of zinc supplements, 42
Lactase, 58
Lacto-ovo-vegetarianism, 16-17
Lactose, in cereals, 100
Lamb's quarters, 95
Lappe, Frances Moore, 18
Laxatives, 93, 151
Lead, 45-46, 113
Leafy greens, 100
Learning disabilities
and mother's smoking, 127
and sugar intake, 66
Lecithin, 39-40
Lee, Royal, 1, 87, 164
Leeks, 152
Lemon juice, 69, 152
Lentils, 100
Let's LIVE, 44, 136
Lettuce, 33, 100, 152
spraying of, 109
Leucine, 16
Levulose, 71
Libby, Alfred, 135-136
Lignin, 100-102
Lime juice, 152
Lipase, 52
Liver
and protein intake, 17
and zinc, 42
Liver tablets, 40-41
Loganberries, 152
Lunch suggestions, 149-150, 159, 163
Lungs, 126
Lysine, 16

McGee, Charles, 164
Magnesium, 40, 121
and bran fiber, 91, 99
sources of, 62, 71, 83

varying content in vegetables, 33
Man Alive You're Half Dead (Munro), 148
Manganese, 42
varying content in vegetables, 33
Mannitol, 122
Maoris of New Zealand, diet of, 31
Marijuana addiction, 132-134
overcoming of, 135-138
Marital problems, and diet, 104-105
Matchan, Don, 128-131
Meal planning
breakfast, 111, 149, 159, 161-162
dinner, 150, 159-160, 163
lunch, 149-150, 159, 163
snacks, 162
Meats
in curative diet, 141-145, 147-151
and drug withdrawal, 135-136
and individual metabolism, 14-15
nutrients in, 15, 41-42
in primitive diet, 25, 30-31
processed, 47
see also Animal protein; Proteins
Media
control of, 165
and eating habits, 75
and smoking, 129
Meditation
and drug withdrawal, 131, 136, 138
and healing, 71
Megavitamins, 133, 136
see also Supplements

Memory improvement, and honey, 69
Menstruation
and iron deficiency, 41
and irritability, 43
Mental disturbance, 136-138
and sugar intake, 123
Mental-emotional problems
see Emotional problems
Mental retardation, and protein intake, 16-17
Metabolism
and alcoholism, 119
and carbohydrate intake, 146
and individual diet, 14-15, 19, 22, 81
Methionine, 16
Methylenechloride, 124
Micronutrients, 33, 38, 41-45, 62-63
Migraine, 155
see also Headaches
Milk
and digestion of cereals, 100